Medical Terminology Quick Learn

The Easiest Guide to Mastering Basic Medical Terminology

Randall A. Simmons, M.Ed., CRCR

ISBN: 978-0-9970874-2-0

10 9 8 7 6 5 4 3 2 1

Visit
quicklearnguides.com
for more information, the latest details and to
inquire about quantity discounts.

Also available:
ICD-10-CM Quick Learn

Welcome to the don't-sweat-it style of learning that cuts to the chase and makes learning fun

Accelerates learning so you can pursue an exciting career in the healthcare field or the medical insurance industry. **Improves efficiency** for anyone who works where medical terminology is used, and anyone who wants to gain a deeper understanding of medical terms.

No long boring lists of words to memorize! **Learn quickly**, no sweat!

You'll analyze fascinating Greek and Latin root words to easily decipher the meanings. Page by page, chapter by chapter, the mysteries are solved, and you'll be able to figure out long alien-sounding medical words that you've never seen before. No sweat!

You'll learn to effortlessly comprehend words like
Cholecystolithiasis
Esophagogastroduodenoscopy
Hysterosalpingography
Thromboendarterectomy

What's inside? 800 medical terms. Exercises with complete answers. Quick Quizzes and Quick Reviews to help you remember. "You've got this!" exercises to build confidence. "Take Note!" tips to help you learn. "It's All Greek [or Latin] to me!" overviews of medical word parts. Clues to help you along. And an Index of medical words and word parts you've learned to use as a reference.

The author brings his unique classroom manner to the printed page, **making learning easy and fun**.

About the author

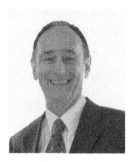

In his three decades of experience in the healthcare reimbursement business, Randall A. Simmons, M.Ed., CRCR, has worked with both providers and payers.

Mr. Simmons holds a Bachelor of Science in psychology, a Master of Education in instructional technology and is a Certified Revenue Cycle Representative.

After gaining more than a decade of experience in the healthcare insurance industry, Mr. Simmons established his own software company and developed proprietary software to process health insurance claims. He has developed computer and internet-based training programs for medical providers as well as for large and small health insurance companies in North America and abroad.

Mr. Simmons has taught in both the academic environment as a college workforce development instructor and at the corporate level in the medical and insurance fields. He is the author of *ICD-10-CM Quick Learn* and has developed numerous handbooks, guides and other teaching tools.

My sincerest thanks to everyone who contributed to this work. A special acknowledgement to Margie Olsen, a gifted illustrator who created the "You've got this!" character. And, a very special acknowledgment and a huge thanks to Karen T. Bartlett for her encouragement, support, editing, design, marketing expertise and much more.

Contents

Continued...

Contents (continued)

How it works

Each lesson in this book is a series of scenarios with multiple choice questions. Hints are everywhere even in the answer choices. It's an open book quiz, so if you're not sure of the answer, just go back and check! To get the most from this **Quick Learn Guide**, it is important to <u>answer the questions on the front of the page, and then turn the page to find the answers</u> (often with extra explanations). This form of interaction will help you learn faster and help you retain the new knowledge.

Front of page

17.2
The gallbladder has two major parts: the bladder and the ducts. Its ducts connect it to the liver and the duodenum. Which disease below refers to an inflammatory problem in the duct?

_____ Cholecystalgia   ✓_____ Cholangiolitis   _____ Cholecystogram

17.3
What if Dr. Sharp's patient has an inflammation of the common bile duct, the big one? This duct is used by the pancreas, the liver, and the gallbladder. What's the name of this disease?

_____ Cholecystogram   _____ Cholangitis   ✓_____ Choledochitis

---

Back of page

17.2
<u>Cholangiolitis</u> is inflammation of the gall bladder duct.

Cholangiolitis has three major word parts: *chol-* refers to bile; *angio-* refers to vessel; *-itis* refers to inflammation. Remember, you've seen the word part, *angio-*, before. Angiitis is the inflammation of a blood or lymph vessel. In this word, the vessel is the smaller bile ducts.

17.3
<u>Choledochitis</u> is inflammation of the common bile duct.

Choledochitis has three major word parts: *chole-* refers to bile; *doch-* refers to duct; and *-itis* refers to inflammation. When *doch-* is combined with *chole-*, it always refers to the largest duct, the common bile duct.

Chapter Quizzes

Each chapter ends with matching exercises or fill in the blank exercises for additional practice. The answers to these exercises are in Appendix A.

NOTE: These quizzes are to give you practice with medical terms. Most chapters have 2 sets of exercises. It is recommended that you complete the first set, wait a few days and then complete the second set. This will help your brain store the information in long term memory.

Sample Matching

Choose the correct match.

_____ 12.1 Surgical excision of part of the lung	A. Thoracentesis
_____ 12.2 Incision into the thyroid cartilage of the larynx	B. Laryngotracheobronchitis
_____ 12.3 A surgical opening into the chest wall	C. Thyrotomy
_____ 12.4 Surgical binding of the pleural layers	D. Pleurodesis
_____ 12.5 Narrowing of the larynx	E. Thoracostomy
_____ 12.6 The softening of the tissue of the voice box	F. Tracheotomy
_____ 12.7 A faster than normal rate of breathing	G. Tachypnea
_____ 12.8 A surgical incision into the trachea	H. Lobectomy
_____ 12.9 A puncture, using a needle, into the chest	I. Laryngostenosis
_____ 12.10 Inflammation of the larynx, the trachea, and the bronchi	J. Laryngomalacia

Sample Fill-in-the-blank

Write-in the correct word from the list below.

12.19 Air pockets in the chest _____

12.20 Swelling of the tissue of the voice box _____

12.21 The act of inserting a tube _____

12.22 Above the glottis _____

You've got this!

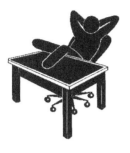

These exercises present you with new medical terms we haven't shown. You will know the parts that make up the medical words. You will see how you understand medical words you've never encountered because now you know the terms that make up the larger words.

Quick Quiz

Quick Quizzes will help you remember information covered previously. You'll find the answers in Appendix A. These exercises are meant to reinforce your new knowledge of medical prefixes, suffixes and definitions.

QUICK QUIZ *(Answers in Appendix A)*	
_____ 7.1 *Hydro-*	*A.* Vein
_____ 7.2 *Vesico-*	*B.* Water or watery like substance
_____ 7.3 *Lipo-*	*C.* Fat tissue
_____ 7.4 *Phlebo-*	*D.* The bladder

Take Note!

Wherever you see the "Take Note!" symbol you will see info as well as tips about medical prefixes, suffixes, terms and learning medical terminology in general.

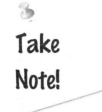

Take Note!

Prefixes are word parts at the beginning of a word.

Suffixes are word parts at the end of words.

Quick Review

Quick Reviews give you a booster shot! Previously learned medical prefixes and suffixes are listed with their definition. Reading these will help you remember the roots.

Quick Review	
Hepato- = liver	**Adeno-** = gland
Osteo- = bone	**Angi-** = blood and lymph vessels
Arthro- = joint	**Blepharo-** = eyelid

CLUE

Clues help you remember previously learned terms and discover the answer to a question.

CLUE

Combine the prefix that means stomach and the suffix that means abnormal flow or discharge!

Word Tour

You'll be amazed at your progress when you work the exercises in the Word Tours. After every five chapters there is a Word Tour that gives you a chance to show off what you've learned. These are review questions on the medical terms you've covered so far. As with the Chapter Quizzes there are two sets of exercises. It is recommended that you complete the first set, wait a few days and then complete the second set. The answers are in Appendix A.

Final Test

The Final Test gives you one last chance to showcase your new knowledge. There are two versions of the final test: Part 1 and Part 2. In Part 1 you are given the definition and you must match it to the term. In Part 2 you are given the term and you must match it to the definition. The answers to the final test are in Appendix A.

It's all Greek [or Latin] to me!

Medical terminology is made of word parts or terms. Most of these terms come from Greek and Latin roots.

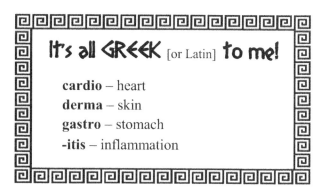

It's all GREEK [or Latin] to me!

cardio – heart
derma – skin
gastro – stomach
-itis – inflammation

Throughout each chapter, when new medical terminology is introduced, whether a prefix, suffix or root word, it is accompanied by a quick reference info box such as the one shown here. These let you know the new terms we will be covering in the coming questions. Of course you'll have scenarios and questions on these new terms to help you learn them. And, as you learn the new terms you will be practicing the terms you previously learned. This method of learning helps you remember.

Index of Word Parts and Words

In Appendix B you will find an index of the medical word parts included in this book and an index of the words you've learned in this book.

Conventions

Medical word parts are shown in *bold italics* as in these examples:

Derma- = skin

-itis = inflammation (so dermatitis is inflammation of the skin.)

NOTE: Certain word parts can appear as prefixes, suffixes or somewhere in the middle of a medical term. A hyphen after the term indicates that it is being used as a prefix in this case. A hyphen before the term indicates that it is being used as a suffix in this case.

Information for instructors

While it is a superior self-learning guide for students on their own, *Medical Terminology Quick Learn* also is an exceptional auxiliary tool for teachers in the classroom environment. Several learning strategies are combined to make this the easiest and most interesting way for students to gain and retain critical knowledge. The approach is informal and friendly with a variety of scenario based practice exercises that keep the student fully engaged. The exercises are followed by immediate feedback. Scenario-based questions add interest and keep the student's attention. Important information is reviewed several times in varying formats including Quick Quizzes and Chapter Quizzes, eliminating the need for rote memorization and repetitiveness utilized in older style textbooks. With the exception of review exercises, students are never presented more than seven questions without receiving feedback in keeping with the rule of thumb known as Miller's law.

In the first five chapters students learn basic medical terms and build the foundation necessary to understand more complex terms. Instructors may choose to use the Word Tour chapters and Final Test as exams, or the questions can form the basis of instructor-generated tests.

This **Quick Learn Guide** can be used in the classroom, assigned as homework, or a combination of the two methods. To help place the terms and information into the student's long-term memory, it is suggested that students concentrate on one chapter at a time. Each chapter reviews and builds upon the important information contained in the prior chapters; a method which has been proven to enhance retention of the material.

Medical Terminology Quick Learn focuses on the "need to know" rather than the "nice to know", giving students plenty of practice using roots, prefixes and suffixes to understand complex medical terminology. This book combines illustrations, a high-level of interaction, and combines repetition with novelty in order to maximize learning.

Information for students

You already know more than you think! Medical terms look difficult because they use Latin and Greek word parts and some are very long. Many are not commonly used in everyday communications. But some you will already be familiar with. And even the long, difficult sounding terms, after you take them apart and learn the secrets, you can easily detect the meaning of what once seemed to be an impossible word.

You may have seen medical terms such as

Cholecystolithiasis
Esophagogastroduodenoscopy
Pancreatoduodenostomy

Words like these are unfamiliar to most of us. Do you want to memorize these words and 997 more? Of course you don't.

Don't let them scare you. This book reveals the secret to identifying and understanding medical terms. You'll be shocked at how many of these words you can learn quickly and simply by applying one small trick you will learn in this book. When you finish this course on medical terminology, you'll not only know new words, but you will also be able to decipher words you have never seen before. Want proof of that? You will prove it to yourself when you work the "You've got this!" exercises at the end of most chapters.

Don't worry if you don't know the answer. Think about the question and choose what you think is the correct answer. Look at the answer choices carefully, they will help you know the correct answer. The questions are not a test. Think of them as a detective game. The purpose of these questions is to help you learn faster. When you read the answers to the questions you will learn more information that will help your medical vocabulary grow.

Who knew you could have fun with medical terminology! Let's get started.

1

Let's Get Started

Let's start by looking at three Greek-based terms that relate to parts of the body.

Look at the first three terms in the list on the right. In this book we use these lists to introduce terms to you. Then you will get lots of practice using them. Before long, they will become second nature to you.

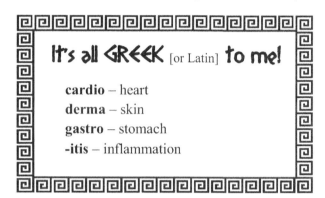

It's all GREEK [or Latin] to me!

cardio – heart
derma – skin
gastro – stomach
-itis – inflammation

1.1
Cardio- is derived from a Greek word, meaning

_____ Stomach   _____ Skin   __X__ Heart

1.2
Derma- is derived from a Greek word, meaning

_____ Stomach   __X__ Skin   _____ Heart

1.3
Gastro- is derived from a Greek word, meaning

__X__ Stomach   _____ Skin   _____ Heart

1.1
Cardio- means <u>heart</u>.

You know the old saying – cold hands, warm cardio!

1.2
Derma- means s<u>kin</u>.

You might say: Beauty is only derma deep!

1.3
Gastro- refers to the <u>stomach</u>!

You can gastro it!

Now you know three medical terms for parts of the body. Here's the magic - by learning one more word part, you will know SIX words.

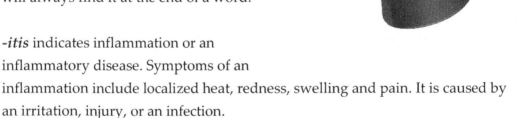

Take this word part: *-itis*. It's a suffix. You will always find it at the end of a word.

-itis indicates inflammation or an inflammatory disease. Symptoms of an inflammation include localized heat, redness, swelling and pain. It is caused by an irritation, injury, or an infection.

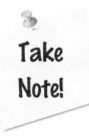

Take Note!

Prefixes are word parts at the beginning of a word.

Suffixes are word parts at the end of words.

1.4

So, if a doctor has a patient whose heart is inflamed, he would diagnose the problem as

CLUE

Now you get to combine two word parts to make a new word – combine a prefix with a suffix!

~~_____~~ Carditis (*cardio-* + *-itis*)
_____ Gastritis (*gastro-* + *-itis*)
_____ Dermatitis (*derma-* + *-itis*)

1.5

What if you notice small blisters on your arm? You may have a problem known to doctors as

_____ Carditis (*cardo-* + *-itis*)
_____ Gastritis (*gastro-* + *-itis*)
~~_____~~ Dermatitis (*derma-* + *-itis*)

1.6

A patient goes to the doctor complaining of pain in his stomach. It's possible that the patient has

_____ Carditis (*cardo-* + *-itis*)
~~_____~~ Gastritis (*gastro-* + *-itis*)
_____ Dermatitis (*derma-* + *-itis*)

Take Note!

Sometimes a t (or other letter) is added to make the word easier to say. For example, the t in derma **t** itis.

1.4

Carditis is an inflammation of the heart.

Cardio- means heart. *-itis* means inflammation. *Cardio-* + *-itis* = carditis.

1.5

Dermatitis is the name for inflammation of the skin.

Derma- means skin. *-itis* means inflammation. *Derma-* + *-itis* = dermatitis.

1.6

Gastritis means inflammation of the stomach.

Gastro- means stomach. If you combine it with *-itis* (inflammation), you have a new word, gastritis.

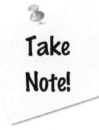

Take Note!

Remember, medical terminology is made of small words put together to make big words.

-itis means inflammation

Cardio- means heart + *-itis* = carditis = inflammation of the heart
Derma- means skin + *-itis* = dermatitis = inflammation of the skin
Gastro- means stomach + *-itis* = gastritis = inflammation of the stomach

When you see a big word, break it down into the little words that make up the big word.

The list on the right shows a few more terms.

You may have heard these words:

HEMOrrhage

HEMOphiliac

HEMOrrhoid

It's all GREEK [or Latin] to me!

arterio – artery
hemo – blood
procto – anus
-rrhage – abnormal or excessive flow or discharge

1.7

What does *hemo-* mean?

_____ Anus   _X_ Blood   _____ Artery

1.8

Which part of the body, does *arterio-* refer to?

_____ Anus   _____ Blood   _X_ Artery

1.9

Another word for *procto-* is

_X_ Anus   _____ Blood   _____ Artery

1.10

If a doctor's diagnosis for a patient is 'hemorrhage,' the patient has

_X_ An abnormal or excessive blood flow or discharge

_____ An inflammation

_____ A severe pain

1.7

Hemo- indicates <u>blood</u>.

Blood flows through the circulatory system.

1.8

Arterio- indicates <u>artery</u>.

The arteries are the blood vessels that carry the blood <u>away</u> from the heart.

1.9

Procto- indicates <u>anus</u>.

Procto- comes from the Greek word proktos, meaning anus or rectum.

1.10

-rrhage indicates <u>an abnormal or excessive flow or discharge</u>.

Hemo- + *-rrhage* = hemorrhage.

Let's take a second look at the word, hemorrhage. It's made up of *hemo-* + *-rrhage*.

Hemo- is a prefix (a prefix is always at the beginning of a word).
-rrhage is a suffix (a suffix is always at the end of a word).

Medical terms are created by combining prefixes and suffixes. As you will see, you can also put word parts in between the prefix and the suffix (more on that later).

The list on the right are some common suffixes.

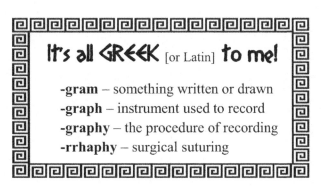

It's all GREEK [or Latin] to me!

-gram – something written or drawn
-graph – instrument used to record
-graphy – the procedure of recording
-rrhaphy – surgical suturing

1.11

If a patient has an abnormal discharge in the stomach, the doctor's diagnosis may be

CLUE Combine the prefix that means stomach and the suffix that means abnormal flow or discharge!

_____ Hemorrhage

__X__ Gastrorrhagia

_____ Gastritis

1.12

What does Doctor Sharp do to stop the hemorrhaging from an artery?

CLUE Start with the prefix that means artery!

__X__ An arteriorrhaphy

_____ A gastrorrhaphy

_____ An arteritis

1.13

What might the doctor do if the patient has gastrorrhagia?

_____ An arteriorrhaphy   __X__ A gastrorrhaphy   _____ An arteritis

1.14

Before text messaging people had to send messages called telegrams. *-gram* is a suffix indicating 'something that is written or drawn'. During an annual examination, a doctor might examine the patient's heart by looking at a recording of the rhythm of the heart. This recording is

_____ An arteriogram   __X__ A cardiogram   _____ A candygram

1.15

Dr. Sharp just x rayed his patient's artery. What's another word for the x-ray?

__X__ An arteriogram   _____ A cardiogram   _____ A candygram

1.11

Gastrorrhagia is a hemorrhage from the stomach.

Gastro- means stomach. *–rrhagia* means an abnormal flow or discharge.
Gastro- + *-rrhagia* = gastrorrhagia.

1.12

Arteriorrhaphy is a surgical suturing of an artery.

(*arterio-* + *-rrhaphy*). *-rrhaphy* indicates surgical suturing. Doctor Sharp might perform an arteriorrhaphy on a patient to stop an artery from hemorrhaging.

You may not have seen *–rrhaphy* previously, but you can still figure out the correct answer by eliminating the other choices. You know *gastro-* refers to the stomach so gastrorrhaphy could not be the correct answer. Likewise, you know *–itis* means inflammation so arteritis could not be correct.

1.13

The doctor might perform a gastrorrhaphy to stop hemorrhaging in the stomach.

(*gastro-* + *-rrhaphy*). He would suture the wound in the stomach.

1.14

A cardiogram (*cardio-* + *-gram*) is the recording of the rhythm of the heart.

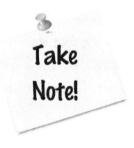

Electrocardiogram is another common word for cardiogram.

Cardio- = heart. *–gram* = a recording.

1.15

An arteriogram is the recording of the blood flow through an artery.

Arterio- refers to the artery. *-gram* refers to the recording of something written or drawn. *Arterio-* + *-gram* = arteriogram.

1.16

The x-ray shows that the patient's artery is inflamed. Dr. Sharp's diagnosis might be

_____ Hemorrhage   ✗ Arteritis   _____ Gastritis

1.17

Doctor Sharp uses a cardiogram to examine characteristics of his patient's heart. What instrument do you think he uses to record this information?

✗ Cardioscope   (Cardiograph)   _____ Cardiomegaly

1.18

Dr. Sharp has a patient with inflammation of the anus. What's this condition called?

CLUE

End with the suffix that means inflammation!

✗ Proctitis
_____ Proctorrhaphy
_____ Proctorrhagia

1.19

What is the term for operating a cardiograph?

CLUE

It's kind of like photography!

_____ Carditis
✗ Cardiography
_____ Arteriography

1.20

What would you call the technique used to produce an arteriogram?

_____ Carditis   _____ Cardiography   ✗ Arteriography

1.16

Arteritis (*arterio- + -itis*) means 'inflammation of an artery.'

An arteriogram might show the inflammation. *Arter-* refers to artery and *–itis* means inflammation.

1.17

A cardiograph (*cardio- + -graph*) is used to record the rhythm of the heart.

-graph is a suffix that indicates an instrument used to record writing or drawing. It can also mean the written or drawn material. Did you notice how similar the suffixes G R A m and G R A p h are? Both refer to writing.

1.18

Proctitis is inflammation of the anus.

Procto- refers to the anus. *-itis* means inflammation. Put them together and you get proctitis (inflammation of the anus).

1.19

Cardiography (*cardio- + -graphy*) refers to the procedure the doctor uses to record the activity of the heart. This technique produces a cardiogram.

1.20

Arteriography (*arterio- + -graphy*) is the name of the technique used to produce a picture of an artery, an arteriogram.

QUICK QUIZ *(Answers in Appendix A)*

1.1 **Cardio-** = _Heart_   1.4 **Procto-** = _anus_

1.2 **Gastro-** = _Stomach_   1.5 **Arterio-** = _artery_

1.3 **Hemo-** = _blood_   1.6 **Derma-** = _skin_

Chapter Quiz (Answers in Appendix A)

Choose the correct match.

A	1.1 Inflammation of the heart	A. Carditis
F	1.2 Surgical suturing of an artery	B. Cardiogram
E	1.3 Excessive flow or discharge in the stomach	C. Cardiograph
B	1.4 Recording of the rhythms of the heart	D. Hemorrhage
D	1.5 Excessive bleeding	E. Gastrorrhagia
C	1.6 An instrument that records rhythms of the heart	F. Arteriorrhaphy
G	1.7 An inflamed artery	G. Arteritis

F	1.8 X-ray of the artery	A. Gastritis
B	1.9 Inflammation of the anus	B. Proctitis
G	1.10 A surgical suturing of the stomach	C. Cardiography
A	1.11 Inflammation of the stomach	D. Dermatitis
C	1.12 Technique of recording the activity of the heart	E. Arteriography
D	1.13 Inflammation of the skin	F. Arteriogram
E	1.14 The technique used to produce an arteriogram	G. Gastrorrhaphy

Write-in the meaning of the term.

1.15 –graphy = the procedure of recording

1.16 -rrhaphy= surgical suturing

1.17 –itis = inflammation

1.18 –graph = instrument used to record

1.19 –rrhage = excessive flow

1.20 –gram = record written in drawn

Write-in the correct word from the list below.

1.21 Surgical suturing of an artery _Arteriorraphy_

1.22 Inflammation of the heart _Carditis_

1.23 An inflamed artery _Arteritis_

1.24 Excessive flow or discharge in the stomach _Gastrorrhagia_

1.25 Excessive bleeding _Hemorrhage_

1.26 Recording of the rhythms of the heart _Cardiography_

1.27 An instrument that records rhythms of the heart _Cardiograph_

1.28 Inflammation of the anus _Proctitis_

1.29 The technique used to produce an arteriogram _Arteriography_

1.30 Inflammation of the stomach _Gastritis_

1.31 X-ray of the artery _Arteriogram_

1.32 Technique of recording the activity of the heart _Cardiogram_

1.33 Inflammation of the skin _Dermatitis_

1.34 A surgical suturing of the stomach _Gastrorrhaphy_

Hemorrhage	Cardiogram	Arteriorrhaphy
Gastrorrhagia	Carditis	Cardiograph
Arteritis	Gastrorrhaphy	Arteriogram
Cardiography	Proctitis	Gastritis
Arteriography	Dermatitis	

2

Some Basic Terms

Let's look at a few more Greek and Latin terms.

It's all GREEK [or Latin] to me!

hepato – liver
-ia – indicates disease or condition
nephro – kidney
pneumo – lungs
pulmonary – lungs

2.1

Have you heard of pneumonia? What does *pneumo-* refer to?

_____ Liver   _____ Kidney   __✓__ Lungs

2.2

What about this word part: *-hepato*? You've might have heard of this disease: hepatitis (*hepat-* + *-itis*). What does *hepato-* mean?

__✓__ Liver   _____ Kidney   _____ Lungs

2.3

Someone who has hepatitis is suffering from:

_____ Excessive bleeding in the liver
__✓__ Inflammation of the liver
_____ Overactivity of the liver

2.1

Pneumo- refers to air or the <u>lungs</u>.

Pneumonia is an inflammation of the lungs caused by bacteria or virus. The suffix *–ia* is Latin for disease or condition. Pneumo comes from a Greek word meaning 'breath.' Pulmonary, from Latin, is also used to refer to the lungs.

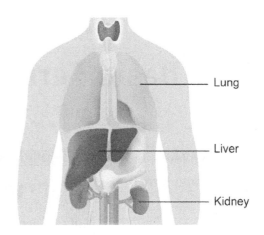

Lung

Liver

Kidney

2.2

Hepato- means <u>liver</u>.

Hepato- comes from a Greek word referring to the liver.

2.3

Hepatitis means <u>inflammation of the liver</u>.

Hepatitis is composed of two word parts: *hepato-* + *-itis*. Remember *-itis* indicates an inflammation. *Hepato-* refers to the liver.

Ready for some new Greek and Latin terms?

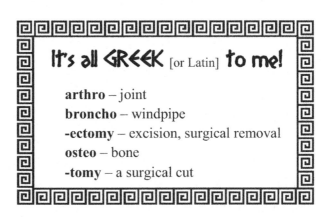

It's all GREEK [or Latin] to me!

arthro – joint
broncho – windpipe
-ectomy – excision, surgical removal
osteo – bone
-tomy – a surgical cut

2.4

Which part of the body does *nephro-* refer to?

_____ Liver   __✗__ Kidney   _____ Lungs

2.5

Dr. Sharp diagnosed his new patient as having inflammation of the lungs. In his notes he wrote

__✗__ Pneumonia   _____ Nephrorrhaphy   _____ Hepatitis

2.6

What if Doctor Sharp performs a surgical suture on the kidney? What procedure would he indicate in his notes?

_____ Pneumonitis   __✗__ Nephrorrhaphy   _____ Gastrorrhagia

2.7

Doctor Sharp's patient has a serious problem with a kidney and the doctor will remove the kidney. Which surgical procedure does he perform?

__✗__ Nephrectomy   _____ Hepatectomy   _____ Gastrectomy

2.8

Later that day, Dr. Sharp has to perform a hepatectomy. What does Dr. Sharp do?

_____ Remove part of the kidney   __✗__ Remove part of the liver
_____ Remove part of the stomach   _____ Remove a section of skin

2.9

When a doctor surgically cuts into a body part, the suffix, *-tomy* (or *–otomy*), is used. For example, Dr. Sharp had a patient with a kidney stone. He had to cut into the kidney to remove the stone. What did he do?

__✗__ Nephrotomy   _____ Hepatotomy   _____ Gastrotomy

2.4

Nephro- refers to the <u>kidneys</u>. It comes from a Greek word meaning kidney.

2.5

<u>Pneumonia</u> is an inflammation of the lungs.

Pneumo- is the Greek word for lungs. *–ia* is Latin for disease. Pneumonia and pneumonitis are both diseases characterized by an inflammation of the lungs.

2.6

<u>Nephrorrhaphy</u> is the name for a surgical suture of the kidney.

Nephro- (meaning kidney) + *-rrhaphy* (meaning surgical suture) gives you nephrorrhaphy, the surgical suturing of the kidney.

2.7

<u>Nephrectomy</u> is the surgical removal of the kidney.

Nephro- means kidney. *-ectomy* indicates the removal of a part by surgery. When you combine *nephro-* and *-ectomy,* you get nephrectomy, the surgical removal of the kidney.

2.8

Hepatectomy means <u>removal of part of the patient's liver</u>.

Hepato- means liver. If you add *hepato-* to *-ectomy,* you have one word that means the surgical removal of part of the liver.

2.9

A surgical cut into the kidney is called a <u>nephrotomy</u> (*nephro-* + *-tomy*).

-tomy indicates a surgical cut. *Nephro-* means the kidney.

2.10

What is the name for removing a part of the stomach?

__✗__ Gastrectomy   _____ Hepatectomy   _____ Nephrectomy

2.11

The doctor's service was nephrotomy. What did the doctor do?

_____ Removed the kidney   *CLUE*

__✗__ Cut into the kidney

_____ Examined the kidney

 Check the Greek/Latin box on page 14!

2.12

Dr. Sharp has diagnosed his patient with osteitis. His patient was suffering from

_____ Hardening of the joint   __✗__ Inflammation of the bone

_____ Excessive bleeding in the windpipe

2.13

Dr. Sharp's next patient has a diagnosis of bronchorrhagia. What's this patient suffering from?

__✗__

_____ Excessive bleeding from the windpipe

_____ Inflammation of the joint

_____ Hardening of the arteries

QUICK QUIZ *(Answers in Appendix A)*

2.1 **Gastro-** = Stomach   2.5 **Pneumo-** = lungs

2.2 **Hemo-** = blood   2.6 **Hepato-** = liver

2.3 **Procto-** = Rectum (anus)   2.7 **Nephro-** = Kidney

2.4 **Arterio-** = artery   2.8 **Derma-** = Skin

2.10

Gastrectomy is the surgical removal of part of the stomach.

Gastro- means stomach. *-ectomy* indicates surgical removal. Put them together and you have gastrectomy, the surgical removal of part of the stomach.

2.11

Nephrotomy means to cut into the kidney.

-tomy indicates to surgically cut into a body part. *-ectomy* looks a lot like *-tomy*, but -ectomy means to remove the part surgically.

2.12

Osteitis is inflammation of the bone.

Osteitis = *oste- + -itis.*
Osteo- refers to bone.
-itis indicates
inflammation. Put them
together and you have
inflammation of the bone.

Take Note!

If osteitis is inflammation of the bone, what do you think arthritis is?
If you said inflammation of the joint, you are correct!

2.13

Bronchorrhagia is excessive bleeding from the windpipe.

(*broncho- + -rrhagia*). *Broncho-* = windpipe. *-rrhagia* = bleeding.

A few more Greek and Latin terms for this chapter.

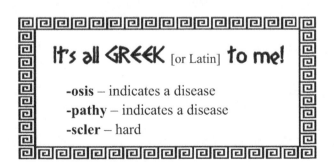

It's all GREEK [or Latin] to me!

-osis – indicates a disease
-pathy – indicates a disease
-scler – hard

2.14

The doctor made an incision into the patient's joint. What's the name of this service?

CLUE

There's a difference between *—ectomy* and *—tomy*!

_____ Arteriorrhaphy   X Arthrotomy   _____ Nephrectomy

2.15

One disease that affects the bones is hardening of the bones. What is the name of this disease?

_____ Osteotomy   _____ Osteitis   X Osteosclerosis

2.16

Dermatosis indicates a disease of the

_____ Head

X Skin

_____ Liver

CLUE

You learned *derma-* on page 1!

2.17

Arthropathy indicates a disease of the

_____ Bone   _____ Artery   X Joint

2.18

You've got this! You're familiar with some new terms now. Let's see how much word power you've developed. Here is a medical term we haven't shown you yet, but you'll be able to decipher its meaning. What does osteoarthritis mean?

(*osteo-* + *arthr-* + *-itis*)

Inflammation in of the junt & of a bone

2.14

Arthrotomy (*arthro-* + *-tomy*) is the name for a surgical cut into the joint.

Arthro- means joint. *-tomy* indicates a surgical incision.

2.15

Osteosclerosis means hardening of the bones (*osteo-* + *scler-* + *-osis*).

Osteo- refers to bone. *Scler-* indicates hard. *-osis* indicates a disease or abnormal condition.

2.16

Dermatosis (*derma-* + *-osis*) is the name for a skin disease.

Derma- means skin. *–osis* indicates a disease.

2.17

Arthropathy is a disease of the joint.

Arthro- refers to the joint. *-pathy* means disease. *Arthro-* + *-pathy* = arthropathy.

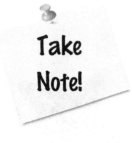

Take Note!

-osis indicates a disease or abnormal condition.
-pathy, like *-osis*, indicates a disease or abnormal condition. As you can see, *-pathy* and *-osis* mean the same thing.
You will come across other pairs of medical terms that mean the same as each other.

2.18

Osteoarthritis is inflammation in the joint and bone.

(*osteo-* + *arthr-* + *-itis*). Osteoarthritis is the most common form of arthritis. Look for the word parts: *osteo-* = bone + *arthro-* = joint + *-itis* = inflammation. Therefore, osteoarthritis is inflammation involving both the joint and the bone.

Chapter Quiz (Answers in Appendix A)

Choose the correct match.

_K_	2.1 Excessive bleeding from the windpipe	A. Arthritis
_A_	2.2 Inflammation of the joints	B. Pneumonia
_H_	2.3 Removal of part of the stomach	C. Osteitis
_J_	2.4 Surgical cut into a joint	D. Nephrorrhaphy
_C_	2.5 Inflammation of the bones	E. Nephrectomy
_B_	2.6 Inflammation of the lungs	F. Dermatosis
_E_	2.7 Removal of part of the liver	G. Hepatectomy
_D_	2.8 Surgical suturing of the kidney	H. Gastrectomy
_F_	2.9 Disease of the skin	I. Nephrotomy
_G_	2.10 Surgical cut into the kidney	J. Arthrotomy
_I_	2.11 Removal of a kidney	K. Bronchorrhagia

Write-in the meaning of the term.

2.12 *Pneumo-* = ___lungs___   2.15 *Arthro-* = ___joint___

2.13 *Hepato-* = ___liver___   2.16 *Nephro-* = ___Kidney___

2.14 *Osteo-* = ___bones___   2.17 *Broncho-* = ___wind pipe___

You've got this! Use your new knowledge to decipher these words.

_B_	2.18 Procedure of x-raying a joint	A. Hepatotomy
_D_	2.19 Procedure for x-raying the windpipe	B. Arthrography
_A_	2.20 Surgical cut into the liver	C. Nephritis
_C_	2.21 Inflammation of the kidneys	D. Bronchography

Write-in the correct word from the list below.

2.22 Removal of part of the stomach _____

2.23 Removal of a kidney _____

2.24 Inflammation of the bones _____

2.25 Surgical cut into the liver _____

2.26 Removal of part of the liver _____

2.27 Surgical suturing of the kidney _____

2.28 Inflammation of the joints _____

2.29 Procedure of x-raying a joint _____

2.30 Inflammation of the lungs _____

2.31 Inflammation of the kidneys _____

2.32 Disease of the skin _____

2.33 Surgical cut into a joint _____

2.34 Procedure for x-raying the windpipe _____

2.35 Excessive bleeding from the windpipe _____

2.36 Surgical cut into the kidney _____

Hepatectomy	Arthritis	Nephrectomy
Hepatotomy	Gastrectomy	Osteitis
Arthrography	Nephrorrhaphy	Nephritis
Bronchography	Pneumonia	Bronchorrhagia
Nephrotomy	Dermatosis	Arthrotomy

3

More Basic Terms

Adeno is a Latin word for gland. It refers to glands including the adrenals (above the kidneys), the thyroid and parathyroid (in the neck), and the lymph nodes and glands. There are several other

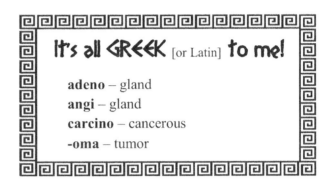

It's all GREEK [or Latin] **to me!**

adeno – gland
angi – gland
carcino – cancerous
-oma – tumor

glands in the body. Most glands produce hormones that control body functions. For instance, the pancreas produces insulin.

Let's look at some problems associated with the glands in the body. With your knowledge of word parts, you will already know most of these.

3.1
What does adenitis refer to?

_____ Hardening of the   _X_ Inflammation of   _____ Disease of the
      gland   the gland   gland

3.2
What does adenosclerosis refer to?

_X_ Hardening of the   _____ Inflammation of   _____ Disease of the
      gland   the gland   gland

3.1
Adenitis is an
<u>inflammation of the
gland</u>, often an
inflammation of the
lymph nodes.

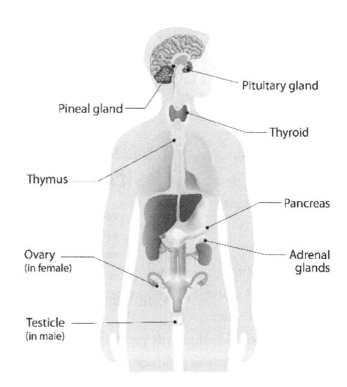

Adenitis has two word
parts: *adeno-* + *-itis*.
Adeno- refers to the
glands. *-itis* indicates
an inflammation.

3.2
Adenosclerosis is the
<u>hardening of a gland</u>.

Adenosclerosis has
three word parts: *adeno-* + *scler-* + *-osis*. *Adeno-* refers to glands. *Scler-* indicates
hard. *-osis* indicates a disease.

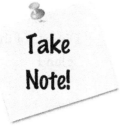

**Take
Note!**

Remember, always look for the little
words that make up the big words.

Quick Review	
Derma- = skin	*Cardio-* = heart
Gastro- = stomach	*Arterio-* = artery

3.3

What does adenopathy mean?

_____ Hardening of the   _____ Inflammation of   ⨉ Disease of the
       gland   the gland   gland

3.4

Dr. Sharp performs an adenectomy. What is he doing?

_____ Cutting into a gland

⨉ Removing a gland

_____ Examining the gland

CLUE

The "ec" in front of
—tomy gives you the
answer!

3.5

Here's a new word part: *-oma*. It is a word ending (suffix) that indicates a tumor.
Dr. Sharp has a patient with osteoma. What condition does the patient have?

⨉ Bone tumor   _____ Liver tumor   _____ Kidney tumor

3.6

Dr. Sharp has to find out what kind of tumor it is. There are several word parts to
describe tumors. If a patient has a cancerous tumor what kind of tumor is it?

_____ Benign   _____ Adenoma   ⨉ Carcinoma

3.7

The patient has hepatocarcinoma.
Where does the patient have a tumor?

_____ Kidney

⨉ Liver

_____ Stomach

CLUE

Carcinoma is the
type of tumor, so
concentrate on
hepato-! See
page 13!

3.3

Adenopathy is a <u>disease of the gland</u>. This often refers to a swelling in the lymph nodes.

Adeno- refers to gland. *-pathy* indicates disease.

3.4

An adenectomy is the <u>surgical removal of a gland</u>.

Adenectomy has two word parts: *adeno-* + *-ectomy*. *Adeno-* refers to glands. *-ectomy* indicates surgically removing a body part.

3.5

Osteoma is <u>bone tumor</u>.

Osteoma is made up of two word parts: *oste-* + *-oma*. *Oste-* refers to the bone. *-oma* indicates a tumor. Dr. Sharp's patient has a bone tumor.

3.6

A <u>carcinoma</u> is a cancerous tumor.

Carcinoma has two word parts: *carcino-* + *-oma*. *Carcino-* refers to cancerous. *-oma* indicates a tumor. Put the two word parts together and you get carcinoma.

3.7

Hepatocarcinoma refers to a tumor in the <u>liver</u>.

As you can see, hepatocarcinoma is a long word. But you know all three word parts: *hepato-* + *carcino-* + *-oma*. *Hepato-* refers to liver. *Carcino-* means cancerous. *-oma* means tumor. The patient has a cancerous tumor in the liver.

Quick Review	
Nephro- = kidney	*Broncho-* = windpipe
Pneumo- = lungs	*Hemo-* = blood

3.8

You've got this! Let's see how much word power you've developed. Here is a medical term we haven't shown you yet, but you'll be able to decipher its meaning. What does gastrocarcinoma mean?

(*gastro-* + *carcino-* + *-oma*)

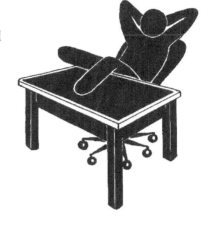

a cancerous tumor in the stomach

3.9

A new patient comes to see Dr. Sharp. The diagnosis is adenocarcinoma. Where is the tumor?

__X__ Gland   _____ Liver   _____ Kidney

3.10

Here's a new word part: *angi-*. Which part of the body does *angi-* refer to?

_____ Stomach   __X__ Blood and Lymph Vessels   _____ Liver

3.11

The patient has angioma. What does the patient have?

__X__ A tumor made up of blood or lymph vessels
_____ Hardening of the blood or lymph vessels
_____ A cancerous blood or lymph vessel

3.12

What is the meaning of angiosclerosis?

_____ A tumor made up of blood or lymph vessels
_____ An inflammation in a blood or lymph vessel
__X__ Hardening of the blood or lymph vessels

3.8

The patient has a <u>cancerous tumor in the stomach</u>.

Gastrocarcinoma is made up of three word parts: *gastro-* + *carcino-* + *-oma*. *Gastro-* refers to stomach. *Carcino-* means cancerous. *-oma* means tumor.

3.9

An adenocarcinoma is a cancerous tumor found in a <u>gland</u>.

Look for the smaller words: *adeno-* + *carcino-* + *-oma*. *Adeno-* refers to glands. *Carcino-* refers to cancerous. *–oma* means tumor.

3.10

Angi- refers to the <u>blood and lymph vessels</u>.

3.11

Angioma is <u>a tumor made up of blood or lymph vessels</u>.

Angioma is composed of two word parts: *angi-* + *-oma*. *Angi-* refers to blood or lymph vessels. *-oma* means tumor.

3.12

Angiosclerosis is a disease characterized by <u>hardening of the blood or lymph vessels</u>.

Angiosclerosis is made up of three word parts: *angio-* + *scler-* + *-osis*. *Angio-* refers to the blood or lymph vessels. *Scler-* means hard. *-osis* indicates disease.

Here's the next list of word parts we will cover in this chapter.

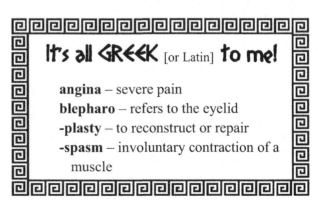

It's all GREEK [or Latin] **to me!**

angina – severe pain
blepharo – refers to the eyelid
-plasty – to reconstruct or repair
-spasm – involuntary contraction of a
  muscle

3.13

The patient has a diagnosis of angiitis. What does the patient hav

_____ A tumor made up of blood or lymph vessels
_____ An inflammation in a blood or lymph vessel
_____ Hardening of the blood or lymph vessels

3.14

Here's a new word part: *-plasty*. It refers to work doctors do when they form, repair, or reconstruct a part of the body. Plastic surgery is a common term for this type of procedure. Dr. Sharp is performing an angioplasty. What is he reconstructing?

_____ The liver   _____ The blood or lymph vessels   _____ The glands

3.15

Dr. Sharp is performing a bronchoplasty. What is he doing?

_____ Repairing the   _____ Reconstructing the   _____ Forming the nose
     lungs   windpipe

3.16

Here's a new word that refers to a part of the body: *blephar-*. What does it mean?

_____ Glands   _____ Lymph vessels   _____ Eyelid

3.17

What does a patient have when Dr. Sharp says the condition is blepharitis?

_____ A nervous tic in   _____ An inflammation of   _____ A cut in the eyelid
     the eyelid   the eyelid

...igiitis is <u>inflammation of the blood or lymph vessels</u>.

Angiitis has two word parts: *angi-* + *-itis*. *Angi-* refers to the blood or lymph vessels. *-itis* indicates an inflammation of a body part.

3.14
Angioplasty is reconstruction of <u>the blood or lymph vessels</u>.

Angioplasty is made up of two word parts: *angi-* + *-plasty*. *Angi-* refers to the blood or lymph vessels. *-plasty* means to reconstruct or repair.

3.15
Bronchoplasty is <u>the reconstruction of the windpipe</u>.

Bronchoplasty has two word parts: *broncho-* + *-plasty*. *Broncho-* refers to the part of the throat that branches into the lungs. *-plasty* indicates surgical reconstruction or repair of a body part.

3.16
Blephar- refers to the <u>eyelid</u>.

3.17
Blepharitis is an <u>inflammation of the eyelid</u>.

Blepharitis is made up of two word parts: *blephar-* + *-itis*. *Blephar-* refers to the eyelid. *-itis* indicates an inflammation.

QUICK QUIZ *(Answers in Appendix A)*

3.1 *Osteo-* = _____.

3.4 *Hepato-* = _____.

3.2 *Broncho-* = _____.

3.5 *-ectomy* = _____.

3.3 *Arthro-* = _____.

3.6 *-tomy* = _____.

3.18

Dr. Sharp had a patient with something in his eye. He had to perform a blepharotomy. What did Dr. Sharp do?

_____ Removed the   _____ Cut into the eyelid   _____ Examined the
     eyelid   eyelid

3.19

Next, Dr. Sharp performed a blepharorrhaphy. What did Dr. Sharp do?

_____ Removed the   _____ Sewed up a cut in the   _____ Cut into the eyelid
     eyelid   eyelid

3.20

Here's a new word part that you might already know: *-spasm*. If your doctor tells you that you have blepharospasm, what do you have?

_____ Uncontrollable   _____ Bleeding from   _____ Inflammation of
     winking of the eyelid   the eyelid   the eyelid

3.21

The doctor performed a cardiorrhaphy. What did the doctor suture?

_____ Head   _____ Blood vessels   _____ Heart

3.22

You've got this! Let's see how well you can use your word power now. What is an angiocardiogram? (*angio-* + *cardio-* + *-gram*)

_____

3.18

Blepharotomy is the procedure of surgically <u>cutting into the eyelid.</u>

Blepharotomy is made up of two words: *blepharo-* + *-tomy*. *Blepharo-* refers to the eyelid. *-tomy* indicates a surgical cut.

3.19

Blepharorrhaphy is <u>sewing up a cut in the eyelid.</u>

Blepharorrhaphy is made up of two words: *blepharo-* + *-rrhaphy*. *Blepharo-* refers to the eyelid. *-rrhaphy* indicates surgically sewing up a body part.

3.20

Blepharospasm is the <u>uncontrollable winking of the eyelid.</u>

Blepharospasm is made up of two words: *blepharo-* + *-spasm*. *Blepharo-* refers to eyelid. *-spasm* refers to the involuntary contraction of a muscle. Sometimes Blepharospasm results in near closure of the eye.

3.21

Cardiorrhaphy is suturing of the <u>heart muscle.</u>

Cardiorrhaphy is made up of two words: *cardio-* + *-rrhaphy*. *Cardio-* refers to the heart. *–rrhaphy* indicates surgically sewing up a body part.

3.22

Angiocardiogram is an <u>x-ray of the heart and its blood vessels.</u>

Angiocardiogram has three word parts: *angio-* + *cardio-* + *-gram*. *Angio-* means blood or lymph vessels. *Cardio-* is heart. *-gram* is a recording.

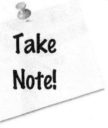

Take Note!

Some medical terms, such as *cardio*, can be a prefix or they can appear in the middle of a word.

3.23

Angina is the name for chest pain. It gets this name because the pain is caused by:

_____ Disease of the heart muscle

_____ Hardening of the blood vessels associated with the heart

_____ Inflammation of the heart

3.24

Dr. Sharp has a patient with adenoma. What's wrong with the patient?

_____ Tumor of the   _____ Tumor of a gland   _____ Involuntary

  lymph vessels   contractions of a gland

3.25

Dr. Sharp had to perform an angiorrhaphy. What did he do?

_____ Sutured a gland   _____ Contained bleeding   _____ Sutured a blood

                               in bony tissue   vessel

3.26

Dr. Sharp's patient has bronchitis. How would you describe this condition?

_____ Inflammation of the bronchial tubes

_____ Inflammation of the eyelid

_____ Disease of the eyelid

3.27

You've got this! Let's see how well you can use your word power now. Dr. Sharp performs a blepharoplasty. What is he doing?
(**blepharo- + -plasty**)

_____

3.23

Angina is caused by <u>hardening of the blood vessels associated with the heart</u>.

Notice the first four letters are *angi-*. Remember *angi-* indicates the blood or lymph vessels. Angina is severe pain that is often accompanied by a choking feeling.

3.24

Adenoma refers to a <u>tumor of a gland</u>.

Adenoma is made up of two word parts: *aden-* refers to gland and *–oma* refers to a tumor. Put them together and you get a tumor of a gland.

3.25

When Dr. Sharp performed an angiorrhaphy he <u>sutured a blood vessel</u>.

Angiorrhaphy is composed of two word parts: *angio-* refers to blood (or lymph) vessels and *–rrhaphy* refers to surgical suturing. Put those word parts together and you get angiorrhaphy, the surgical suturing of a blood vessel.

3.26

Bronchitis is <u>inflammation of the bronchial tubes.</u>

Bronchitis is made up of two word parts: *bronch-* which refers to the bronchial tubes and *-itis* which means inflammation.

3.27

Blepharoplasty is <u>repairing or reforming the eyelid</u>.

Blepharoplasty is made up of two word parts: *blepharo-* refers to eyelid and *–plasty* means to repair or reform a body part. Another way to say it is blepharoplasty is plastic surgery on the eyelid.

Chapter Quiz 1 (Answers in Appendix A)

Choose the correct match.

_____ 3.1 Involuntary muscle contraction of eyelid	A. Blepharitis
_____ 3.2 Repairing the windpipe	B. Blepharospasm
_____ 3.3 Inflammation of the blood or lymph vessel	C. Blepharotomy
_____ 3.4 Sewing up the eyelid	D. Angiitis
_____ 3.5 Inflammation of the gland	E. Blepharoplasty
_____ 3.6 Hardening of the gland	F. Bronchoplasty
_____ 3.7 Inflammation of the eyelid	G. Adenitis
_____ 3.8 Surgically cutting into the eyelid	H. Adenosclerosis
_____ 3.9 Repairing the eyelid	I. Blepharorrhaphy

You've got this! Use your new knowledge to decipher these words.

_____ 3.10 Angiectomy	A. Any disease of blood or lymph vessels
_____ 3.11 Angiospasm	B. Uncontrolled contraction of blood vessels
_____ 3.12 Angiosis	C. Excision of a blood vessel
_____ 3.13 Angiocarditis	D. Inflammation of the heart and it's blood vessels
_____ 3.14 Angiogram	E. The machine used to x-ray the blood vessels
_____ 3.15 Angiocardiography	F. The procedure of x-raying the heart and blood vessels
_____ 3.16 Angiograph	G. An x-ray of the blood vessels
_____ 3.17 Angiography	H. Involuntary muscle contraction of windpipe
_____ 3.18 Bronchospasm	I. The procedure of x-raying the blood vessels

Write-in the correct word from the list below.

3.19 Hardening of the blood or lymph vessels _____

3.20 Disease of a gland_____

3.21 Tumor of the blood or lymph vessel _____

3.22 Cancerous tumor of the liver _____

3.23 Surgical reconstruction of a blood or lymph vessel _____

3.24 Cancerous tumor of the gland _____

3.25 Surgical removal of a gland_____

3.26 Tumor of the bone _____

3.27 Cancerous tumor of the stomach _____

3.28 Severe pain in the chest area _____

Angina	Osteoma	Gastrocarcinoma
Angioplasty	Adenocarcinoma	Adenopathy
Adenectomy	Angiosclerosis	Angioma
Hepatocarcinoma		

Chapter Quiz 2 (Answers in Appendix A)

Choose the correct match.

_____ 3.29 Cancerous tumor of the stomach	A. Adenopathy
_____ 3.30 Severe pain in the chest area	B. Angioma
_____ 3.31 Tumor of the bone	C. Hepatocarcinoma
_____ 3.32 Cancerous tumor of the liver	D. Angioplasty
_____ 3.33 Disease of a gland	E. Angiosclerosis
_____ 3.34 Cancerous tumor of the gland	F. Adenectomy
_____ 3.35 Surgical removal of a gland	G. Osteoma
_____ 3.36 Surgical reconstruction of a blood or lymph vessel	H. Gastrocarcinoma
_____ 3.37 Tumor of the blood or lymph vessel	I. Angina
_____ 3.38 Hardening of the blood or lymph vessels	J. Adenocarcinoma

You've got this! Use your new knowledge to decipher these words.

_____ 3.39 Proctorrhaphy	A. Suturing of the heart muscle
_____ 3.40 Nephropathy	B. Suture of the windpipe
_____ 3.41 Hepatopathy	C. Excessive flow of blood from a bone
_____ 3.42 Cardiorrhaphy	D. Bleeding from the rectum
_____ 3.43 Bronchorrhaphy	E. Disease of the liver
_____ 3.44 Dermatorrhagia	F. Suturing of the rectum
_____ 3.45 Osteorrhagia	G. Disease of the kidney
_____ 3.46 Proctorrhagia	H. Hemorrhage into or from the skin

Write-in the correct word from the list below.

3.47 Hardening of the gland _____

3.48 Inflammation of the eyelid _____

3.49 Involuntary muscle contraction of the eyelid _____

3.50 Surgically cutting into the eyelid _____

3.51 Inflammation of a blood or lymph vessel _____

3.52 Surgical repair or reconstruction of the eyelid _____

3.53 Surgical repair of the windpipe _____

3.54 Inflammation of the gland _____

3.55 Involuntary muscle contraction of windpipe _____

3.56 Surgically sewing up the eyelid _____

Bronchospasm	Adenitis	Blepharorrhaphy
Blepharitis	Adenosclerosis	Bronchoplasty
Angiitis	Blepharoplasty	Blepharospasm
Blepharotomy		

4

Additional Vocabulary

Here's a few of the Greek and
Latin terms we will cover in
this chapter.

It's all GREEK [or Latin] **to me!**

-algia – pain
cephal – refers to the head
ot – indicates the ear
-scope – instrument used to examine
-scopy – looking at something

4.1

The term *cephal-* refers to the head. Let's say you have a terrible headache. What
would Dr. Sharp call it?

_____ Cephalitis   _____ Cephalalgia   _____ Cephaloma

4.2

Here's a long word, but you know
all the parts: cephalhematoma.
What does it mean?

CLUE

Cephal- + hema- + -oma

_____ Loss of control of muscles due to brain damage
_____ Collection of blood beneath the scalp
_____ Malignant tumor of the skin

4.3

Let's take another look at *–algia*. What does arthralgia refer to?

_____ Pain in the chest   _____ Pain in the stomach   _____ Pain in the joints

4.1

Cephalalgia is the term for a headache.

Cephal- refers to the head. Whenever you see it, you know the person has a problem associated with the head. *-algia* indicates pain or disease. *Cephal-* + *-algia* is a diagnosis, meaning headache.

4.2

Cephalhematoma is a collection of blood beneath the scalp.

Cephal- refers to the head. *Hema-* refers to blood. *-oma* refers to a mass (of blood in this case). Cephalhematoma is usually found in a newborn. It is caused by excessive pressure at birth.

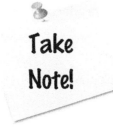

Take Note!

Have you ever had a black eye?

A black eye is the collection of blood near the skin. It is caused by trauma. Doctors refer to it as a hematoma. *Hema-* refers to blood and *–oma* refers to a tumor or mass. A hematoma can occur anywhere on the body. It is the result of blood escaping from a blood vessel, often due to a trauma.

4.3

Arthralgia is pain in the joints.

Remember *arthro-*? *Arthro-* refers to the joints. *–algia* means pain. Put them together and you get arthralgia, pain in the joints.

Quick Review	
-ia- = disase or condition	*-osis-* = disease or condition
-pathy- = disease or condition	**All three of these terms indicate a disease or condition.**

4.4

What does otalgia refer to?

_____ Pain in the bone   _____ Pain in the lungs   _____ Pain in the ear

4.5

A lot of people are sensitive because they think their ears are too big. Some people have surgery to reconstruct their ears. What do you call this surgery?

_____ Otitis   _____ Otoplasty   _____ Otoscopy

4.6

Have you ever looked through a telescope? When you wanted to see the stars better? Well, then, you already know what kind of an instrument an otoscope is. What do doctors use an otoscope for?

_____ To examine the outer ear, eardrum, and middle ear
_____ To record sound waves
_____ To clean the ear

4.7

Dr. Sharp has a new patient. The diagnosis is bronchorrhagia. The service is bronchoscopy. What did the doctor do?

_____ Examined the windpipe
_____ Looked at a gland
_____ Reconstructed a blood vessel

CLUE

broncho- gives you the solution! See page 11!

4.8

Dr. Sharp has a patient with an earache. He wants to look at the ear. What will he do?

_____ Gastroscopy   _____ Arthroscopy   _____ Otoscopy

4.4

Otalgia is <u>pain in the ear</u>, an earache.

"Ot" did you say? *Ot-* indicates ear. *-algia* indicates pain. *Ot-* + *-algia* = earache.

4.5

Reconstruction of the ear is <u>otoplasty</u>.

Ot- refers to ear. *-plasty* refers to the surgical procedure for forming or reconstructing a part of the body. When you see *-plasty*, think "plasty" surgery!

Take Note!   *Do you remember that **osteo-** refers to bone? It looks a lot like **oto-**. But notice the "s" and "e" in **osteo-**.*

4.6

An otoscope is <u>an instrument used to examine the outer ear, eardrum, and middle ear</u>.

-scope is a suffix used to indicate an instrument used for observing or detecting. Think microSCOPE or teleSCOPE. An otoSCOPE is used to examine the ear!

4.7

Dr. Sharp did a bronchoscopy to <u>exam the windpipe</u>.

Remember *broncho-*? It refers to the windpipe, the part of your throat that branches into the lungs. Bronchoscopy is looking at the inside of the windpipe with a special instrument. *- scopy* (scope + Y) is viewing, seeing, or examining using some kind of scope.

4.8

Examining the inside of the ear is called <u>otoscopy</u>.

Ot- + *-scopy*. *Ot-* refers to the ear. *-scopy* refers to looking at something.

Here's a few more terms that we will add to your knowledgebase.

It's all GREEK [or Latin] to me!

colo – refers to the colon
hystero – refers to the uterus
myo – refers to the muscle
-stomy – a surgical opening

4.9

Dr. Sharp has a patient who is afraid he has a stomach ulcer. Dr. Sharp decides to look inside his patient's stomach. What is Dr. Sharp doing?

_____ Gastroscopy   _____ Arthroscopy   _____ Otoscopy

4.10

Colo- is Latin for colon, a part of the large intestines. The patient has a diagnosis of colitis. What is wrong with the patient?

_____ Disease of the   _____ Inflammation of   _____ Bleeding in the
       colon   the colon   colon

4.11

A patient has a very bad case of colitis. Dr. Sharp decides he must create a surgical opening in the colon. In this way, he can allow material to exit the body without passing through the colon. This will give the colon time to heal. What is this procedure called?

_____ Colostomy   _____ Colonoscopy   _____ Colpectomy

4.12

Dr. Sharp has a patient in a coma. He must make a surgical opening into the stomach to feed the patient. What's this operation called?

_____ Nephrostomy   _____ Gastrotomy   _____ Gastrostomy

4.9

The best response is <u>gastroscopy</u>.

Remember *gastro-*? It refers to the stomach. *Gastro-* + *-scopy* means the examination of the stomach. When a doctor looks inside your stomach using a long tube with a visual piece, he is performing a gastroscopy.

4.10

Colitis is <u>inflammation of the colon</u>.

Remember *-itis*? It means an inflammation. *Col-* + *-itis* means inflammation of the colon. That's colitis!

4.11

A <u>colostomy</u> is a surgical opening in the colon.

Colo- + *-stomy*. *Colo-* refers to colon. *–stomy* indicates a surgical opening.

4.12

A surgical opening into the stomach is a <u>gastrostomy</u>.

Take Note!

Be careful! –stomy looks a lot like –tomy. –stomy indicates a surgical opening. –tomy indicates an incision (cut).
A surgical opening (–stomy) is usually performed to allow doctors to artificially feed the patient or to allow materials to leave the body, as in a colostomy.

QUICK QUIZ *(Answers in Appendix A)*

4.1 *Cephalo-* = _____.   4.5 *–scopy* = _____.

4.2 *–algia* = _____.   4.6 *Colo-* = _____.

4.3 *Ot-* = _____.   4.7 *–stomy* = _____.

4.4 *–scope* = _____.   4.8 *Hemo-* = _____.

4.13

Let's learn another word part. *Hystero-* refers to the uterus, also known as the womb. Dr. Sharp has a patient who is having problems. He decides to make an incision into her womb to explore her problem. What procedure does he perform?

_____ Hysterectomy   _____ Hysterotomy   _____ Hysteroscopy

4.14

What is a hysteroscopy?

_____ Examination where the doctor looks inside the womb
_____ The removal of the womb
_____ Surgical opening in the womb

4.15

The next procedure is a hysterectomy. What did the doctor do?

_____ Removed the   _____ Cut into the   _____ Examined the womb
         womb   womb

4.16

Here's a new word part: *myo-*. Which body part does *myo-* refer to:

_____ The head   _____ The glands   _____ The muscle

4.17

The next patient has myalgia. How would you describe this condition?

CLUE

Break the word into its parts:
myo- and *-algia.*

_____ Tumor of the muscles
_____ Aching muscles
_____ Charlie horse

4.13

A <u>hysterotomy</u> is a surgical cut into the womb.

Don't forget *-tomy* means a surgical incision. When you add *-tomy* to *hystero-*, you get hysterotomy.

4.14

An hysteroscopy is <u>an examination where the doctor looks inside the womb</u>.

Don't forget *-scopy*. Think of telescope. *-scopy* means to examine something, often visually. The doctor uses an instrument that allows him to see inside.

4.15

Hysterectomy is the removal of the womb.

-ectomy is a word part that indicates the surgical removal of a part of the body. *Hystero-* refers to the womb.

4.16

Myo- refers to <u>the muscle</u>.

Myo- is a word part from Greek that means muscles. "My O My O - What big muscles you have!"

4.17

Myalgia is <u>aching muscles</u>.

My- refers to muscles; *-algia* indicates pain, or aching. *My-* + *-algia* indicates aching muscles. If you've had the flu, you know what myalgia feels like.

Let's add a couple more terms to our medical vocabulary.

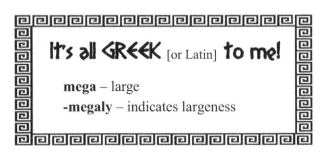

It's all GREEK [or Latin] to me!

mega – large
-megaly – indicates largeness

4.18

Have you ever heard the word part, mega? It means large. *Megaly-* is a Greek word part used to indicate largeness. A body part that is enlarged or too big is not healthy. The patient has a diagnosis of cardiomegaly. What is wrong?

_____ The head is enlarged
_____ The heart is enlarged
_____ The colon is enlarged

Try out your word power! The next three exercises are some words we haven't shown you yet, but you know all or most of their word parts. Use your word power to figure out what they mean.

4.19

You've got this! Here's a long medical term:
cardiomyopathy (*Cardio-* + *myo-* + *-pathy*)
Use your word power to decipher the meaning.

_____

4.20

You've got this! What's the meaning of this medical term?
Gastrocolitis (*Gastro-* + *colo-* + *-itis*)

_____

4.21

You've got this! *Sigmoid-* refers to part of the colon, so, what's the meaning of this medical term? Proctosigmoidoscopy (*Procto-* + *sigmoid-* + *-scopy*)

_____

4.18

Cardiomegaly refers to an <u>enlarged heart</u>.

Cardiomegaly is made up of two word parts: *cardio-* + *-megaly*. *Cardio-* refers to the heart. *-megaly* indicates large. Put *cardio-* and *-megaly* together and you get cardiomegaly.

4.19

Cardiomyopathy means <u>disease of the heart muscle</u>.

It is a long word. Let's break it into its three word parts. *Cardio-* refers to the heart. *Myo-* refers to the muscle. *-pathy* indicates disease.

Put these three word parts together and you get cardiomyopathy - a disease of the muscles of the heart.

4.20

Gastrocolitis is <u>inflammation of the stomach and colon</u>.

Gastrocolitis is made up of 3 word parts: *gastro-* + *colo-* + *-itis*. *Gastro-* refers to the stomach. *Colo-* refers to the colon. *-itis* indicates an inflammation.

4.21

Proctosigmoidoscopy is the <u>visual examination of the colon and rectum</u>.

Proctosigmoidoscopy is made up of 3 word parts. *Procto-* + *sigmoid-* + *-scopy*. *Procto-* refers to the anus. *Sigmoid-* refers to a part of the colon. *-scopy* indicates a visual examination.

Quick Review	
Hepato- = liver	*Adeno-* = gland
Osteo- = bone	*Angi-* = blood and lymph vessels
Arthro- = joint	*Blepharo-* = eyelid
-oma = tumor	*-spasm* = involuntary contraction of a muscle

Chapter Quiz 1 (Answers in Appendix A)

Choose the correct match.

_____ 4.1 Visual exam of the inside of the windpipe	A. Colitis
_____ 4.2 Aching muscles	B. Arthralgia
_____ 4.3 Enlarged heart	C. Bronchoscopy
_____ 4.4 Aching joints	D. Myalgia
_____ 4.5 Visual exam of the inside of the stomach	E. Cardiomegaly
_____ 4.6 Inflammation of the colon	F. Gastrocolitis
_____ 4.7 Headache	G. Cephalalgia
_____ 4.8 Disease of the muscle of the heart	H. Cardiomyopathy
_____ 4.9 Inflammation of the stomach and colon	I. Gastroscopy
_____ 4.10 Pain in the ear	J. Otalgia

You've got this! Use your new knowledge to decipher these words.

_____ 4.11 Otitis	A. Hardening of the bones of the ear
_____ 4.12 Ototomy	B. A disease of the muscle
_____ 4.13 Arthroscopy	C. Incision into the ear
_____ 4.14 Otosclerosis	D. Inflammation of the ear
_____ 4.15 Myopathy	E. A disease of the head or brain
_____ 4.16 Myorrhaphy	F. Surgical connection between the colon and the rectum
_____ 4.17 Myosclerosis	G. Hardening of the muscle
_____ 4.18 Cephalopathy	H. Visual exam of the inside of the joint
_____ 4.19 Colonoscopy	I. Examination of the colon with a scope
_____ 4.20 Coloproctostomy	J. Suture of the muscle

Write-in the correct word from the list below.

4.21 Visual exam of the inside of the womb _____

4.22 Surgical opening into the colon _____

4.23 Instrument used to examine the ear _____

4.24 Visual exam of the inside of the colon and rectum _____

4.25 Visual exam of the inside of the ear _____

4.26 Removal of the womb _____

4.27 Surgical opening into the stomach _____

4.28 Surgical cut into the womb _____

4.29 Reconstruction of the ear _____

4.30 A collection of blood beneath the scalp _____

Cephalhematoma	Proctosigmoidoscopy	Otoplasty
Colostomy	Hysteroscopy	Otoscopy
Otoscope	Gastrostomy	Hysterectomy
Hysterotomy		

Chapter Quiz 2 (Answers in Appendix A)

Choose the correct match.

_____ 4.31 Reconstruction of the ear	A. Hysteroscopy
_____ 4.32 Visual exam of the inside of the colon and rectum	B. Colostomy
_____ 4.33 Collection of blood beneath the scalp	C. Otoscope
_____ 4.34 Surgical opening into the colon	D. Proctosigmoidoscopy
_____ 4.35 Instrument used to examine the ear	E. Otoscopy
_____ 4.36 Surgical opening into the stomach	F. Hysterectomy
_____ 4.37 Removal of the womb	G. Gastrostomy
_____ 4.38 Visual exam of the inside of the womb	H. Hysterotomy
_____ 4.39 Visual exam of the inside of the ear	I. Otoplasty
_____ 4.40 Surgical cut into the womb	J. Cephalhematoma

You've got this! Use your new knowledge to decipher these words.

_____ 4.41 Colotomy	A. Pain in the colon
_____ 4.42 Colonopathy	B. Disease of the bone
_____ 4.43 Colorrhaphy	C. X-ray of a joint
_____ 4.44 Colonalgia	D. Incision of colon
_____ 4.45 Arthrogram	E. Suture of the colon
_____ 4.46 Bronchogram	F. Any disease of the colon
_____ 4.47 Ostectomy	G. Excision of part of the bone
_____ 4.48 Osteopathy	H. X-ray of the windpipe

Write-in the correct word from the list below.

4.49 Inflammation of the colon _____

4.50 Pain in the ear _____

4.51 Visual exam of the inside of the windpipe _____

4.52 Inflammation of the ear _____

4.53 Enlarged heart _____

4.54 Visual exam of the inside of the joint _____

4.55 Headache _____

4.56 Disease of the muscle of the heart _____

4.57 Visual exam of the inside of the stomach _____

4.58 Aching joints _____

Gastroscopy	Cephalalgia	Cardiomyopathy
Colitis	Bronchoscopy	Arthralgia
Cardiomegaly	Otitis	Arthroscopy
Otalgia		

5

Building A Larger Vocabulary

There are still a few Greek and Latin names for body parts we haven't talked about. Let's look at some more.

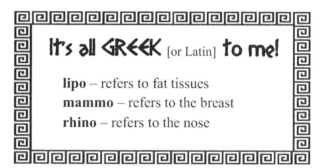

It's all GREEK [or Latin] to me!

lipo – refers to fat tissues
mammo – refers to the breast
rhino – refers to the nose

5.1

For example, we haven't talked about noses, yet. One well-known animal uses this Greek word part. Which word part refers to noses?

_____ *Lipo-*   _____ *Mammo-*   _____ *Rhino-*

5.2

Which word refers to breast?

_____ *Lipo-*   _____ *Mammo-*   _____ *Rhino-*

5.3

The last word refers to fat. Which word part is it?

_____ *Lipo-*   _____ *Mammo-*   _____ *Rhino-*

5.4

Dr. Sharp performs a lipectomy. The patient's diagnosis is lipoma. How do you describe this condition?

_____ Enlarged nose   _____ Enlarged breasts   _____ Harmless tumor made up of fat cells

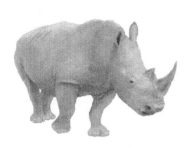

5.1
Rhino- refers to the nose.

How do you think the rhinoceros got its name? Ever seen a rhinoceros? They have very big noses! (well, they have a big horn on their nose)

5.2
Mammo- refers to the breast!

Notice how similar it is to Momma.

5.3
Lipo- refers to fat tissues.

You can remember *lipo-*, it rhymes with hippo, and it means fat.

5.4
Lipoma is the name of a harmless tumor composed of fat cells.

Lipoma is composed of two words: *lipo- + -oma. Lipo-* refers to fat cells. *-oma* indicates a tumor.

QUICK QUIZ *(Answers in Appendix A)*

5.1 *Ot-* = _____.

5.2 *Myo-* = _____.

5.3 *Hystero-* = _____.

5.4 *Cephalo-* = _____.

5.5 *Adeno-* = _____.

5.6 *Angi-* = _____.

5.7 *Arthro-* = _____.

5.8 *Blepharo-* = _____.

Quick Review	
Colo- = colon	*Hyster-* = womb or uterus
Myo- = muscle	*-algia* = pain or aching

5.5
What did the doctor do when he performed the lipectomy?

_____ Made a surgical incision into the fat cells
_____ Removed the fat cells
_____ Examined the fat cells

5.6
The patient wants plastic surgery on his nose. The doctor will perform:

_____ A mammoplasty   _____ A rhinoplasty   _____ A rhinotomy

5.7
Dr. Sharp performs an operation. The service is a mammoplasty. What did Dr. Sharp do?

_____ Reconstructed an   _____ Removed a fat   _____ Reconstructed a
    eyelid   cell   breast

5.8
Jonny Goodhealth had such a bad cold he went to Dr. Sharp for help. His diagnosis was rhinitis. What was wrong with Jonny?

_____ Lungs were inflamed
_____ A disease caused by an African animal
_____ Inner lining of nose was inflamed

5.9
Some doctors suggest that women over the age of 40 should have a mammogram regularly. What is a mammogram?

_____ Instrument to record the fat tissue in the body
_____ X-ray of the soft tissue in the breast
_____ Technique for recording the breath moving through the nose

5.5

Lipectomy is the <u>removal of fat cells.</u>

Lipectomy is composed of two word parts: *lipo-* + *-ectomy*. *Lipo-* refers to fat cells. *-ectomy* refers to a surgical procedure for removing a part of the body.

5.6

<u>Rhinoplasty</u> is surgery that reconstructs one's nose.

Rhino- refers to nose. *-plasty* indicates surgery that forms or reconstructs a body part.

5.7

Mammoplasty is surgery to <u>reconstruct a breast</u>.

Think momma! Mammoplasty is the surgical procedure for reforming the breast. *Mammo-* refers to the breast. *-plasty* indicates a surgical procedure that reconstructs or reforms a body part.

5.8

Rhinitis is the <u>inflammation of the inner lining of the nose</u>. It is often caused by a bad cold.

Rhinitis is composed of two word parts: *rhino-* + *-itis*. Remember *-itis*? It indicates an inflammation. *Rhino-* refers to nose.

5.9

A mammogram is an <u>x-ray of the soft tissue of the breast</u>.

Mammo- refers to the breast. *-gram* refers to a recording of something. Put them together and you get mammogram.

Here's two more terms you'll need to know.

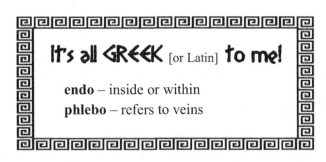

It's all GREEK [or Latin] to me!

endo – inside or within
phlebo – refers to veins

5.10

Let's learn a new word part! *Phlebo-* refers to a part of the body. It's Greek for vein, the blood vessels that carry blood to the heart. You are working with a patient who as a diagnosis of phlebitis. What condition does the patient have?

_____ Enlarged veins

_____ Inflammation of the veins

_____ A condition that causes dogs to itch

5.11

If Dr. Sharp wants to draw blood from someone, he may perform a phlebotomy. What is he doing?

CLUE

Note that "ec" is not in front of *–tomy*!

_____ Removing a vein

_____ Surgically cutting into a vein

_____ Suturing a vein

5.12

Here's a word part you may see often, *endo-*. It means inward or within. What does endocarditis mean?

_____ Enlargement of the inner lining of the uterus

_____ Tumor inside the breast

_____ Inflammation of the membrane lining the inside of the heart

5.13

Now try this word: endoscopy. What does endoscopy mean?

_____ Visual examination of the inside of a body cavity

_____ Recording of the inside of the colon

_____ Removal of the inside the womb

5.14

You've got this! Use your word power to figure out what this term means: Endophlebitis.

(*endo-* + *phleb-* + *-itis*)

5.10

Phlebitis is <u>inflammation of the veins</u>.

Remember *-itis*? It means an inflammation. *Phleb-* + *-itis* means inflammation of the veins. Phlebitis usually occurs in the legs.

5.11

A phlebotomy is <u>surgically cutting into a vein</u>.

Phlebo- + *-tomy*. *Phlebo-* refers to the vein. *-tomy* indicates a surgical incision. A phlebotomy is commonly done to draw blood.

5.12

Endocarditis is <u>inflammation of the membrane lining the inside of the heart</u>.

Endocarditis is a long word. Find the 3 little words that make it up and you can more easily find its meaning: *endo-* + *card-* + *-itis*. *Endo-* means inside. *Card-* refers to heart. *-itis* is an inflammation.

5.13

Endoscopy is a <u>visual examination of the inside of a body cavity</u>.

Endoscopy is made up of two word parts: *endo-* + *-scopy*. *Endo-* means inside. *-scopy* means to see, to look, to view, or to examine.

5.14

Endophlebitis is <u>inflammation of the inside lining of a vein</u>.

endo- + *phleb-* + *-itis*. *Endo-* means inside. *Phleb-* refers to vein. *-itis* indicates an inflammation.

Here's the list of words we are going to cover next.

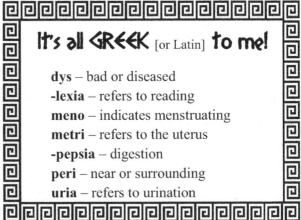

It's all GREEK [or Latin] **to me!**

dys – bad or diseased
-lexia – refers to reading
meno – indicates menstruating
metri – refers to the uterus
-pepsia – digestion
peri – near or surrounding
uria – refers to urination

5.15

The patient has an inflammation of the inner lining of the sac surrounding the heart. What condition does the patient have?

CLUE

Remember to break the words into their parts! This word has four parts!

_____ Myocarditis
_____ Endopericarditis
_____ Endometriosis

5.16

The diagnosis indicates that the inner lining of the uterus is diseased. What is the diagnosis?

_____ Endomyofibrosis _____ Endophlebitis _____ Endometriosis

5.17

Here's a prefix you may see frequently, **Dys-**. It comes from a Greek word meaning diseased, difficult, or bad. Which word means bad digestion or upset stomach?

_____ Dyspepsia _____ Dysmenorrhea _____ Dysuria

5.18

Which word means a difficult or painful menstruation?

_____ Dyspepsia _____ Dysmenorrhea _____ Dysuria

5.19

Which word means painful or difficult urination?

_____ Dyspepsia _____ Dysmenorrhea _____ Dysuria

5.20

The medical term for reading difficulty is

_____ Dyspepsia _____ Dyslexia _____ Dysuria

5.15

Endopericarditis is an inflammation of the inner lining of the pericardium.

Endo- is a word part that means inner. *Peri-* means near or surrounding. Pericardium is the sac surrounding the heart muscle. *-itis* indicates an inflammation.

5.16

Endometriosis is the disease of the inner membrane of the uterus.

Break these long words into their small word parts. *Endo-* = inner, *metri-* refers to the uterus. *-osis* indicates diseased.

5.17

Dyspepsia is an upset stomach.

Dyspepsia is composed of two word parts: *dys-* + *-pepsia*. *Dys-* means bad or diseased. *-pepsia* means digestion. Put them together: you get dyspepsia, an upset stomach.

5.18

Dysmenorrhea is difficult or painful menstruation.

Dysmenorrhea is made up of 3 word parts: *dys-* + *meno-* + *-rrhea*. *Dys-* indicates bad. *Meno-* is derived from the the Greek word meaning month. It indicates menstruating (a woman's monthly period). *-rrhea* indicates a discharge.

5.19

Dysuria means painful or difficult urination.

Dysuria is made up of two word parts: *dys-* + *-uria*. *Dys-* means difficult or bad. *-uria* refers to urination or the urinary tract.

5.20

Dyslexia is the name for reading difficulty.

Dyslexia is made up of 2 words: *dys-* + *-lexia*. *Dys-* means difficult or bad. *-lexia* comes from a Greek word meaning speech.

This list of words may appear daunting, but don't worry – we are going to cover all of these words so you'll know them before long.

It's all GREEK [or Latin] **to me!**

-**centesis** – puncture with a needle
duodeno – refers to small intestines
entero – refers to small intestines
-**iasis** – indicates disease
-**lith** – stones, such as kidney stones
myel – refers to bone marrow
pore – a tiny opening
uro – refers to urine or urinary tract

5.21
What word indicates a disease of the kidneys & urinary tract?

_____ Uroarthritis   _____ Uronephrosis   _____ Uropathy

5.22
What is the medical term for the procedure of recording the elements in a patient's urine?

_____ Urobilin   _____ Urodynamics   _____ Urography

5.23
Which of the following diagnoses is NOT a disease of the intestines?

_____ Gastroenteritis   _____ Gastrohepatitis   _____ Gastroduodenitis

5.24
The patient has a diagnosis of kidney stones. What has the doctor written on the chart to indicate kidney stones?

_____ Hepatocarcinoma   _____ Cephaloma   _____ Nephrolithiasis

5.25
Dr. Sharp's patient has osteoarthritis. Under services the doctor wrote arthrocentesis. What did Dr. Sharp do?

_____ X-rayed the artery
_____ Removed fluid from the joint to identify chemicals present
_____ Reconstructed the ear

5.21

Uronephrosis is a disease that affects the kidneys and the urinary tract.

Uronephrosis is made up of 3 words. *Uro-* + *nephro-* + *-osis*. *Uro-* refers to the urinary tract. *Nephro-* refers to the kidneys. *-osis* indicates disease.

5.22

Urography is the procedure used to record the elements that make up a patient's urine. For instance, a doctor could find too much sugar in the urine.

Urography is made up of two word parts: *uro-* + *-graphy*. *Uro-* refers to the urine. *-graphy* refers to the technique for recording something.

5.23

Gastrohepatitis is an inflammation of the stomach and liver.

Gastro- = stomach. *Hepa-* = liver. *–itis* = inflammation.

The other two words refer to the intestines. *Entero-* is a word part that refers to the intestines, especially the small intestines. *Duodeno-* is a word part that refers to a portion of the small intestine, starting at the lower end of the stomach. *Gastro-* + *entero-* + *-itis*. *Gastro-* + *duodeno-* + *-itis*. Both of these words refer to an inflammation in the intestines and the stomach.

5.24

Nephrolithiasis means kidney stone.

It's made up of three word parts: *Nephro-* + *lith-* + *-iasis*. Remember the word for kidney? *Nephro-* means kidney. *Lith-* is from the Greek word for stone. *-iasis* indicates disease.

5.25

Arthrocentesis is the name of a procedure for using a needle to remove fluid from the joints. Doctors use this fluid to find out what chemicals and microorganisms are present.

Arthrocentesis has two parts: *arthro-* refers to joint. *-centesis* refers to a puncture with a hollow needle.

5.26

A pore is a tiny opening. Your skin has pores. If you see a claim for osteoporosis, what condition does the patient have?

_____ Hardening of the inner ear
_____ Loss of bony tissue, causing fragile bones
_____ Condition in which the glands become soft

5.27

For the next patient, the diagnosis is infection of the bone and bone marrow. What's the medical term for this disease?

_____ Osteosclerosis   _____ Otitis interna   _____ Osteomyelitis

5.28

Dr. Sharp has a new patient. The diagnosis is nephrosis. The service is hemodialysis. What did the doctor do?

_____ Removed wastes and impurities from the blood with a special machine
_____ Examined the blood around the kidneys
_____ Made a surgical opening on the artery leading to the kidneys

5.29

Dr. Sharp takes an x-ray of part of the urinary tract. What is the x-ray called?

_____ An enterogram   _____ A mammogram   _____ A urogram

5.30

If Dr. Sharp makes a surgical incision into a breast, what is the procedure called?

_____ A mammogram   _____ A mammotomy   _____ A mammectomy

5.31

You've got this! Use your word power to figure out what this medical term means: Enterospasm. (*entero* + *spasm*)

_____

5.26
Osteoporosis is the name of a condition in which <u>tiny openings in the bone make the bone fragile</u>. Then they easily break.

Remember *osteo-*? It refers to bone. Osteoporosis is made up of three word parts: *Osteo-* + *pore-* + *-osis*. *-osis*, as you know, indicates disease. Pore is a tiny opening.

5.27
<u>Osteomyelitis</u> is the infection of the bone and bone marrow.

Osteo- refers to bone. Osteomyelitis is made up of three word parts: *osteo-* + *myel-* + *-itis*. *-itis* indicates inflammation. *Myel-* refers to the bone marrow.

5.28
Hemodialysis is the <u>procedure for removing wastes and impurities from the blood</u>.

Remember *hemo-* refers to blood.

5.29
A <u>urogram</u> is an x-ray of part of the urinary tract.

Uro- indicates the urinary tract. *-gram* indicates an x-ray. Put them together and you get a urogram, an x-ray of the urinary tract.

If *uro-* means the urinary tract and *-pathy* indicates disease, what do you think the term for a disease of the urinary tract is?
Answer: Uropathy! (*uro-* + *-pathy*)

5.30
When a doctor makes a surgical incision into the breast it is called a <u>mammotomy</u>.

Remember, *mammo-* refers to breast and *–tomy* means an incision.

5.31
A diagnosis of enterospasm is <u>irregular or painful movement of the intestines</u>.

Entero- refers to the intestines. *–spasm* is any kind of irregular movement of a muscle.

Chapter Quiz 1 (Answers in Appendix A)

Choose the correct match.

_____ 5.1 The sac surrounding the heart	A. Lipectomy
_____ 5.2 Inflammation of the membrane inside the nose	B. Rhinoplasty
_____ 5.3 Harmless tumor made of fat tissue	C. Phlebitis
_____ 5.4 X-ray of the soft tissue of the breast	D. Mammogram
_____ 5.5 Removal of waste products from the blood	E. Mammotomy
_____ 5.6 Removal of fat tissue	F. Lipoma
_____ 5.7 Reconstruction of the nose	G. Pericardium
_____ 5.8 Upset stomach	H. Hemodialysis
_____ 5.9 Inflammation of the vein	I. Rhinitis
_____ 5.10 A surgical incision into the breast	J. Dyspepsia

You've got this! Use your new knowledge to decipher these words.

_____ 5.11 Enteropathy	A. Any disease of the nose
_____ 5.12 Rhinologist	B. Hardening of the vein
_____ 5.13 Rhinopathy	C. A disease of the intestines
_____ 5.14 Phlebectomy	D. Someone who specializes in diseases of the nose
_____ 5.15 Phlebalgia	E. Inflammation of the stomach and portion of small intestines by the stomach
_____ 5.16 Phlebosclerosis	F. An excision of a vein or part of a vein
_____ 5.17 Gastroduodenitis	G. The condition of accumulating fat cells in the body
_____ 5.18 Liposis	H. A surgical suturing of a vein
_____ 5.19 Phleborrhagia	I. Bleeding from a vein
_____ 5.20 Phleborrhaphy	J. Pain arising from a vein

Write-in the correct word from the list below.

5.21 Painful menstruation _____

5.22 Removal of fluid from the joint _____

5.23 Fragile bones caused by tiny pores in tissue _____

5.24 Reconstruction of the breast _____

5.25 Inflammation of the membrane inside the uterus _____

5.26 Infection of the bone & bone marrow _____

5.27 Surgical incision into the vein _____

5.28 Any disease that affects the urinary tract _____

5.29 Kidney stones _____

5.30 Inflammation of the stomach and
        portion of small intestines by the stomach _____

Gastroduodenitis	Osteomyelitis	Endometriosis
Osteoporosis	Phlebotomy	Arthrocentesis
Dysmenorrhea	Nephrolithiasis	Mammoplasty
Uropathy		

Chapter Quiz 2 (Answers in Appendix A)

Choose the correct match.

_____ 5.31 Painful menstruation	A. Dysmenorrhea
_____ 5.32 Kidney stones	B. Uropathy
_____ 5.33 Reconstruction of the breast	C. Arthrocentesis
_____ 5.34 Inflammation of stomach and portion of small intestines by the stomach	D. Osteoporosis
_____ 5.35 Fragile bones caused by tiny pores in tissue	E. Mammoplasty
_____ 5.36 Removal of fluid from the joint	F. Endometriosis
_____ 5.37 Surgical incision into the vein	G. Osteomyelitis
_____ 5.38 Inflammation of the membrane inside the uterus	H. Phlebotomy
_____ 5.39 Infection of the bone & bone marrow	I. Nephrolithiasis
_____ 5.40 Any disease that affects the urinary tract	J. Gastroduodenitis

You've got this! Use your new knowledge to decipher these words.

_____ 5.41 Lipoarthritis	A. Removal of the breast
_____ 5.42 Mammectomy	B. Repair of a vein
_____ 5.43 Mammalgia	C. Inflammation of fatty tissues of joints
_____ 5.44 Rhinorrhagia	D. Examination of the nose using an instrument
_____ 5.45 Phleboplasty	E. Incision of the nose
_____ 5.46 Rhinoscope	F. Bleeding from the nose
_____ 5.47 Rhinoscopy	G. Pain in the breast
_____ 5.48 Rhinotomy	H. Instrument used to examine the nose

Write-in the correct word from the list below.

5.49 Removal of fat tissue _____

5.50 Reconstruction of the nose _____

5.51 Inflammation of the vein _____

5.52 X-ray of the soft tissue of the breast _____

5.53 Upset stomach _____

5.54 A surgical incision into the breast _____

5.55 Harmless tumor made of fat tissue _____

5.56 The sac surrounding the heart _____

5.57 Removal of waste products from the blood _____

5.58 Inflammation of the membrane inside the nose _____

Lipoma	Mammogram	Hemodialysis
Phlebitis	Rhinoplasty	Pericardium
Rhinitis	Dyspepsia	Lipectomy
Mammotomy		

Word Tour 1

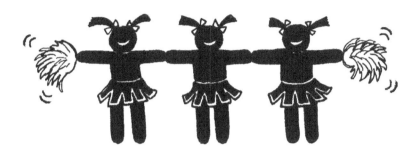

Congratulations! You've made it to the first review. How are you feeling? Take a moment to relax and pat yourself on the back.

Then, when you're ready, forge ahead to these review exercises. Working through these exercises will help you remember the things you've learned so far.

The questions are organized into two parts. You can work them one page at a time and check your answers with each page, or challenge yourself and check your answers after each part.

So, take a moment, then grab your pencil and get started!

NOTES...

Word Tour 1

Part 1 (Answers in Appendix A)

Match the definitions to the terms.

_____ 1.1 Cancerous tumor in the gland	A. Adenocarcinoma
_____ 1.2 Visual exam inside of the windpipe	B. Arteriosclerosis
_____ 1.3 Surgical opening in the colon to allow materials to pass outside	C. Proctosigmoidoscopy
_____ 1.4 Hardening of the artery	D. Dyspepsia
_____ 1.5 Visual exam of the colon and rectum	E. Cephalalgia
_____ 1.6 Headache	F. Angina
_____ 1.7 Fragile bones, easily breakable	G. Angioma
_____ 1.8 Reconstruction of the ear	H. Otoplasty
_____ 1.9 Harmless tumor made of blood vessels	I. Osteoporosis
_____ 1.10 Visual examination of the stomach	J. Bronchoscopy
_____ 1.11 Severe pain	K. Colostomy
_____ 1.12 Upset stomach	L. Gastroscopy

Write-in the meaning of the term.

1.13 *Derma-* = _____   1.16 *Cardio-* = _____

1.14 *Procto-* = _____   1.17 *Pneumo-* = _____

1.15 *Arterio-* = _____   1.18 *Hepato-* = _____

Match the definitions to the terms.

_____ 1.19 Removal of fat tissue   A. Arteriography

_____ 1.20 Reconstruction of the breast   B. Endometriosis

_____ 1.21 Surgical incision into the joint   C. Mammoplasty

_____ 1.22 Inflammation of the inner lining of the   D. Arthrotomy
           womb or uterus

_____ 1.23 Inflammation of the liver   E. Hepatitis

_____ 1.24 Removal of the waste products from the   F. Nephrolithiasis
           blood

_____ 1.25 Hardening of the bones   G. Hemodialysis

_____ 1.26 Tumor made up of fat tissue   H. Lipectomy

_____ 1.27 Procedure for taking an x-ray of the flow   I. Lipoma
           of blood through the artery

_____ 1.28 Removal of the uterus (or womb)   J. Osteosclerosis

_____ 1.29 Kidney stones   K. Hysterectomy

_____ 1.30 Inflammation of the skin   L. Dermatitis

Write-in the meaning of the term.

1.31 *Arthro-* = _____   1.34 *Hemo-* = _____

1.32 *Broncho-* = _____   1.35 *Adeno-* = _____

1.33 *Nephro-* = _____   1.36 *Angi-* = _____

Match the definitions to the terms.

_____ 1.37 Inflammation of the inner lining of the sac surrounding the heart | A. Adenitis

_____ 1.38 Visual exam of the uterus (womb) | B. Osteomyelitis

_____ 1.39 Inflammation of the bone and bone marrow | C. Bronchospasm

_____ 1.40 Muscle contraction in the windpipe | D. Arthralgia

_____ 1.41 Removal of the kidney | E. Hemorrhage

_____ 1.42 Inflammation of the gland | F. Endopericarditis

_____ 1.43 Aching joints | G. Angiocardiogram

_____ 1.44 Reconstruction of the eyelid | H. Blepharoplasty

_____ 1.45 Difficulty reading | I. Dyslexia

_____ 1.46 Excessive bleeding | J. Osteoarthritis

_____ 1.47 Inflammation of the joints (most common type) | K. Blepharitis

_____ 1.48 Recording of the flow of blood through blood vessels of heart | L. Nephrectomy

_____ 1.49 Inflammation of the eyelid | M. Hysteroscopy

Write-in the meaning of the term.

1.50 *-rrhage* = _____   1.53 *–ectomy* = _____

1.51 *–gram* – _____   1.54 *-scler* = _____

1.52 *–ia* = _____   1.55 *–tomy* = _____

Match the definitions to the terms.

_____ 1.56 Difficult or painful urination	A. Endocarditis
_____ 1.57 Visual exam of the inside of a body cavity	B. Mammogram
_____ 1.58 Inflammation of inner lining of the heart	C. Dysmenorrhea
_____ 1.59 Reconstruction of the joint	D. Dysuria
_____ 1.60 Removal of the fluid from the joint using a hollow needle	E. Endoscopy
_____ 1.61 Enlarged heart	F. Otitis
_____ 1.62 Disease affecting the kidney and the urinary tract	G. Arthrocentesis
_____ 1.63 Surgical opening into the stomach, usually for artificial feeding	H. Gastroduodenitis
_____ 1.64 Inflammation of the stomach and portion of small intestine next to the stomach	I. Cardiomyopathy
_____ 1.65 X-ray of the soft tissue of the breast	J. Arthroplasty
_____ 1.66 Inflammation of the ear	K. Cardiomegaly
_____ 1.67 Difficult or painful menstruation	L. Gastrostomy
_____ 1.68 Disease of the muscle of the heart	M. Uronephrosis

Write-in the meaning of the term.

1.69 –*osis* = _____   1.72 –*scope* = _____

1.70 –*oma* = _____   1.73 –*stomy* = _____

1.71 –*plasty* = _____   1.74 –*megaly* = _____

Word Tour 1
Part 2 (Answers in Appendix A)

Match the terms to the definitions.

_____ 1.1 Proctosigmoidoscopy	A. Cancerous tumor in the gland
_____ 1.2 Adenocarcinoma	B. Visual examination of the stomach
_____ 1.3 Colostomy	C. Upset stomach
_____ 1.4 Cephalalgia	D. Visual exam of the inside of the windpipe
_____ 1.5 Bronchoscopy	E. Reconstruction of the breast
_____ 1.6 Otoplasty	F. Surgical opening in the colon to allow materials to pass outside
_____ 1.7 Osteoporosis	G. Harmless tumor made up of blood vessels
_____ 1.8 Arteriosclerosis	H. Reconstruction of the ear
_____ 1.9 Angioma	I. Fragile bones, easily breakable
_____ 1.10 Dyspepsia	J. Headache
_____ 1.11 Gastroscopy	K. Hardening of the artery
_____ 1.12 Mammoplasty	L. Visual exam of the colon and rectum

Write-in the meaning of the term.

1.13 *Rhino-* = _____   1.15 *Myel-* = _____

1.14 **Entero-** = _____   1.16 *Phlebo-* = _____

Match the terms to the definitions.

_____ 1.17 Hemodialysis	A. Inflammation of the skin
_____ 1.18 Hepatitis	B. Inflammation of the inner lining of the womb or uterus
_____ 1.19 Angina	C. Removal of the waste products from the blood
_____ 1.20 Lipectomy	D. Removal of the uterus (or womb)
_____ 1.21 Endometriosis	E. Inflammation of the liver
_____ 1.22 Arthrotomy	F. Inflammation of the bone and bone marrow
_____ 1.23 Nephrolithiasis	G. Visual exam of the uterus (womb)
_____ 1.24 Hysteroscopy	H. Tumor made up of fat tissue
_____ 1.25 Hysterectomy	I. Removal of fat tissue
_____ 1.26 Dermatitis	J. Kidney stones
_____ 1.27 Lipoma	K. Surgical incision into the joint
_____ 1.28 Osteomyelitis	L. Severe pain

Write-in the meaning of the term.

1.29 *Cephal-* = _____   1.32 *Lith-* = _____

1.30 *Myo-* = _____   1.33 *Lipo-* = _____

1.31 *Dys-* = _____   1.34 *Hystero-* = _____

Match the terms to the definitions.

_____ 1.35 Osteosclerosis

A. Recording of the flow of blood through the blood vessels of the heart

_____ 1.36 Endopericarditis

B. Inflammation of the joints (most common type)

_____ 1.37 Arteriography

C. Enlarged heart

_____ 1.38 Dyslexia

D. Aching joints

_____ 1.39 Adenitis

E. Excessive bleeding

_____ 1.40 Blepharoplasty

F. Removal of the kidney

_____ 1.41 Nephrectomy

G. Reconstruction of the eyelid

_____ 1.42 Angiocardiogram

H. Difficulty reading

_____ 1.43 Arthralgia

I. Muscle contraction in the windpipe

_____ 1.44 Osteoarthritis

J. Procedure for taking an x-ray of the flow of blood through the artery

_____ 1.45 Bronchospasm

K. Hardening of the bones

_____ 1.46 Hemorrhage

L. Inflammation of the inner lining of the sac surrounding the heart

_____ 1.47 Cardiomegaly

M. Inflammation of the gland

Write-in the meaning of the term.

1.48 –pepsia = _____

1.51 –scopy = _____

1.49 –iasis = _____

1.52 –algia = _____

1.50 –centesis = _____

1.53 –lexia = _____

Match the terms to the definitions.

_____ 1.54 Arthroplasty	A. Surgical opening into the stomach, usually for artificial feeding
_____ 1.55 Blepharitis	B. Difficult or painful menstruation
_____ 1.56 Uronephrosis	C. Visual exam of the inside of a body cavity
_____ 1.57 Arthrocentesis	D. Difficult or painful urination
_____ 1.58 Gastrostomy	E. Disease affecting the kidney and urinary tract
_____ 1.59 Dysuria	F. Inflammation of the ear
_____ 1.60 Endocarditis	G. Disease of the muscle of the heart
_____ 1.61 Endoscopy	H. Inflammation of the stomach and a portion of the small intestine next to the stomach
_____ 1.62 Cardiomyopathy	I. Removal of the fluid from the joint using a hollow needle
_____ 1.63 Mammogram	J. Inflammation of the eyelid
_____ 1.64 Otitis	K. Inflammation of the inner lining of the heart
_____ 1.65 Gastroduodenitis	L. Reconstruction of the joint
_____ 1.66 Dysmenorrhea	M. X-ray of the soft tissue of the breast

6

The Urinary System, Part 1: Urologist Talk: Cystolithotomy and other easy terms

Three parts of the urinary system are the bladder (stores urine), ureter (transports urine from kidneys to bladder), and urethra (transports urine from bladder to release).

It's all GREEK [or Latin] to me!

cyst – refers to the bladder
-lapaxy – to empty out
-ologist – person who studies a
   subject

6.1

An urologist is a medical doctor who works with:

_____ Organs associated with nerves

_____ Organs in the digestive tract

_____ Organs in the urinary tract

6.2

Let's look at the body parts associated with the urinary tract. Which part of the urinary tract stores urine?

_____ Kidney

_____ Bladder

_____ Ureter

6.3

Which part of the urinary tract carries urine from the kidney to the bladder?

_____ Kidney

_____ Bladder

_____ Ureter

6.1

An urologist works with diseases that affect the <u>body parts in the urinary tract</u>.

A clue is **Uro-**, the first part of urologist. **Uro-** is the Greek word for urine. **-ologist** is the person who studies or works on a subject.

6.2

The <u>bladder</u> is the body part along the urinary tract that stores urine.

6.3

The <u>ureters</u> are those long narrow tubes between the kidneys and the bladder. They carry the urine to its next stop.

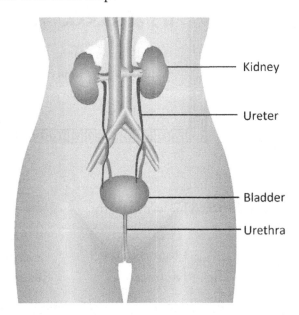

QUICK QUIZ *(Answers in Appendix A)*

_____ 6.1 **Dys-**	**A.** Surrounding
_____ 6.2 **Duodeno-**	**B.** Refers to the intestines, especially the small intestines
_____ 6.3 **Entero-**	**C.** Refers to a portion of the small intestine starting at the lower end of the stomach
_____ 6.4 **Peri-**	**D.** Diseased, difficult, or bad

6.4

While you're looking at the urinary tract, what is the name of the canal that carries the urine to its final destination -- discharge from the body.

_____ Ureter   _____ Urethra   _____ Kidney

6.5

If the kidneys are not working properly, all of the urea may not be sent to the bladder. Some may be absorbed in the blood. A patient with too much urea in the blood may have headaches and nausea. The patient may even go into a coma. When urea is absorbed in the blood, the condition is called

_____ Uremia   _____ Nephritis   _____ Ureter

6.6

The doctor saw a patient the other day whose kidneys are not working properly. As a result, she has too much protein in her urine. What is the diagnosis?

_____ Uremia   _____ Proteinuria   _____ Proteinase

6.7

Sometimes a problem in the urinary tract is caused by an infection in the prostate or vagina. The bacteria may travel up the urinary tract. Dr. Sharp saw a patient, Mr. S. Pete, who was having a burning sensation every time he urinated. His diagnosis was cystitis. What condition is this?

_____ His kidneys are   _____ His bladder is   _____ His ureter is
      infected   infected   swollen

Quick Review	
Entero- = intestines	_Lith-_ = stone(s)
Myel- = bone marrow	_-centesis_ = puncture with a hollow needle

6.4

The <u>urethra</u> is the canal from which we release urine from our bodies.

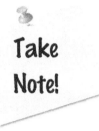

Take Note!

Urethra is from a Greek word meaning to urinate. Notice some words that refer to urine or body parts whose main purpose is to transport urine start with *ur-*.

6.5

<u>Uremia</u> is a condition where the patient has too much urea in the blood.

Urea is a waste product that the kidneys normally send to the bladder to remove it from the body.

6.6

A person with <u>proteinuria</u> has too much protein in the urine.

Proteinuria is a condition usually caused by kidney disease. Break the word into its parts: The first part of proteinuria is protein; the second part is *-uria*. Remember, *ur-* signifies urine.

6.7

Cystitis (*Cyst-* + *-itis*) is the <u>inflammation of the bladder</u>.

Cyst- is often used to refer to the bladder. A cyst is a pouch that contains liquid. The bladder is a pouch that often contains liquid!

Quick Review	
Rhino- = nose	*Lipo-* = fat
Mammo- = breast	*Phleb-* = vein
Endo- = inside or within	*Peri-* = near or around
Dys- = diseased, or difficult, or bad	*Uro-* = refers to the urinary tract

6.8

Mr. Pete's infection kept getting worse. Dr. Sharp decided to x-ray the bladder and the canal below the bladder to identify the problem. What is the procedure called?

_____ Cystolithotomy   _____ Urethrocystography   _____ Ureterolithotomy

6.9

After looking at the x-ray Dr. Sharp decided to get a biopsy of the tissue in the bladder. To get a sample of the unhealthy tissue, he had to perform a

_____ Cystolithotomy   _____ Cystectomy   _____ Cystotomy

6.10

Poor Mr. Pete's bladder just keeps getting worse. Finally, the doctor had to remove most of the bladder. This procedure is called a

_____ Cystolithotomy   _____ Cystectomy   _____ Cystotomy

6.11

Just yesterday, Ms. Rockefellow came to see Dr. Sharp. She was having severe pains in her abdomen. It turned out the problem was stones in her bladder. What did the doctor do to correct her problem?

_____ Cystography   _____ Cystolithotomy   _____ Nephrolithiasis

6.12

A year later Ms. Rockefellow had stones in the tubes that connect the kidneys and the bladder? Which disease describes her problem?

_____ Nephrolithiasis
_____ Ureterolithiasis
_____ Cystolithiasis

CLUE

The key here is the name of the tubes that connect the kidneys and the bladder! Look at the illustration on page 80!

6.8

Urethrocystography is the procedure of x-raying the bladder and the canal below the bladder.

Urethro- = the urethra, the canal below the bladder used to release urine. *Cysto-* = the bladder. *-graphy* is the x-ray technique. Put these word parts together and you have the technique (*-graphy*) of x-raying the bladder (*cysto-*) and the urethra (*urethra-*).

6.9

Dr. Sharp must perform a cystotomy (cut into the bladder), to retrieve the tissue for the biopsy.

Break the word into parts to find its meaning: *cyst-* = bladder and *-tomy* = cut into.

6.10

When a doctor cuts out the bladder, s/he is performing a cystectomy.

Break the word into parts to easily find its meaning: Cystectomy = *cyst-* + *-ectomy* = bladder + cut out. Don't confuse CystECTOMY with CystOTOMY. *-ectomy* means to cut out; *-tomy* means to cut into.

6.11

To remove stones from the bladder, a doctor performs a cystolithotomy.

Break the word apart to see its meaning: *cyst-* = bladder; *lith-* = stone; *-tomy* = surgical cut into. Put the separate meanings together and you get a surgical cut into the bladder to remove stones.

6.12

When someone has stones in the ureter (the canal that connects the kidneys and the bladder), the disease is called ureterolithiasis.

Uretero- = ureter; *lith-* = stones; *-iasis* = disease or condition.

6.13

Dr. Sharp recommended that Ms. Rockefellow have an operation to remove the stones in the ureter. What procedure did he recommend?

_____ Nephrolithotomy   _____ Cystolithotomy   _____ Ureterolithotomy

6.14

Dr. Sharp also uses an endoscope to destroy stones in the bladder or ureter. When he uses an endoscope, what is the operation called?

_____ Catheterization   _____ Litholapaxy   _____ Fulguration

6.15

How about a new word? At the bottom of the bladder is a triangular shaped area between the two openings of the ureters and the urethra. What is the name of this area?

_____ Trigone   _____ Transurethral   _____ Anastomosis

6.16

Ms. Trey came to see Dr. Sharp complaining of frequent and painful urination. After examining Ms. Trey, Dr. Sharp found that the trigone was severely infected. What was his diagnosis?

_____ Cystitis   _____ Trigone   _____ Trigonitis

6.17

Mr. S. Topper came to see Dr. Sharp. He was unable to urinate. He had been experiencing pain when he urinated for quite some time. Dr. Sharp found that not only his trigone but also his urethra was infected. What is the diagnosis?

_____ Urethropexy   _____ Urethrotrigonitis   _____ Urethrocystography

6.13

To remove the stones in the ureter, a doctor might recommend <u>ureterolithotomy</u>.

That is a surgical incision (*-tomy*) to remove the stones (*lith-*) from the ureter (*uretero-*).

6.14

<u>Litholapaxy</u> uses an endoscope to destroy stones in the bladder or ureter.

The clue is *litho-* which means stone. *–lapaxy* means to empty out. Litholapaxy is an operation using a cystoscope. The doctor pushes an instrument through the scope that picks up and crushes the stones. Next he removes this instrument and uses a metal tube to irrigate the bladder and flush out the stones.

6.15

The <u>trigone</u> is the triangular area at the bottom of the bladder.

Trigone is the old Greek word for triangle - the shape of this area. Did you notice TRIgone and TRIangular have similar word parts?

6.16

When the trigone is infected or inflamed, the name of the condition is <u>trigonitis</u>.

Trigon- = trigone; *-itis* = inflammation. Don't forget the trigon is at the bottom of the bladder.

6.17

It's a long word but it's a big infection. <u>Urethrotrigonitis</u> is the word for an infection of the urethra and the trigone (the bottom of the bladder).

Try to break a big word into its parts. Find the little words you know: *urethra-* (urethra) + *trigon-* (the base of the bladder) + *-itis* (infection).

Here's some more terms we
will cover in this chapter.

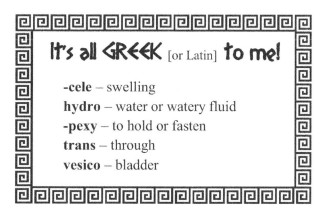

It's all GREEK [or Latin] **to me!**

-cele – swelling
hydro – water or watery fluid
-pexy – to hold or fasten
trans – through
vesico – bladder

6.18

To help Mr. S. Topper, Dr. Sharp inserted a small tube (a catheter) through his
urethra and into the bladder to remove the urine. He also used this tube to wash
out the bladder and urethra. What is this procedure called?

_____ Catheterization   _____ Urethrocystography   _____ Ureterolithiasis

6.19

Ms. Homan came to see the doctor, complaining -- when she coughed or sneezed,
her bladder leaked. This happens when the urethra is not in the normal position.
The doctor explained the procedure: He fixes the urethra in place so that it stays
in its normal position. What is the name of this procedure?

_____ Urethropexy   _____ Transurethral surgery   _____ Anastomosis

6.20

Ms. Bulge is feeling really bad. After examining her, Dr. Sharp took a urogram. It
showed a swelling in the ureters by the opening to the bladder. What is his
diagnosis?

_____ Ureterolithiasis   _____ Hydronephrosis   _____ Ureterocele

6.18

Catheter + ization = the procedure of inserting the catheter. A catheter is a small tube used to open up a closed body channel or to maintain an opening in a body channel.

A body channel might be the urethra or an artery or vein. In this case, the swollen bladder closed the normal opening. The doctor inserted a catheter to reopen the channel.

6.19

During urethropexy the doctor quite literally fixes or fastens the urethra to the wall of the vagina with sutures.

If you break urethropexy into its two parts, you can see the meaning of the word: *urethro-* refers to the urethra; *-pexy* means to hold or fasten. In this operation, the doctor fastens the urethra to the vagina wall.

6.20

Ureterocele describes a swelling of the wall of the ureter at the opening into the bladder.

If you break ureterocele into its parts, you have *uretero-* which indicates the ureter is affected + *-cele* which means swelling.

QUICK QUIZ *(Answers in Appendix A)*

_____ 6.5 Urologist	*A.* The body part along the urinary tract that stores urine
_____ 6.6 Bladder	*B.* The canal that carries the urine to its final destination -- discharge from the body
_____ 6.7 Ureter	*C.* Medical doctor who works with body parts in the urinary tract.
_____ 6.8 Urethra	*D.* Long narrow tubes between the kidneys and the bladder

6.21

Because of the swelling, the urine created in the kidneys was not flowing into the bladder. It was backing up in the kidneys - a condition very damaging to the kidney. What is the name of this condition?

CLUE

Look at the prefixes! Urine is a fluid. Now look at the rest of the word parts.

_____ Nephroureterectomy   _____ Hydronephrosis   _____ Hydroureter

6.22

Of course, since the urine is backed up at the end of the ureter, where it flows into the bladder, the ureters are also filled with urine. This condition is called

_____ Hydroureter   _____ Hydronephrosis   _____ Nephroureterectomy

6.23

If hydronephrosis and hydroureter are not identified early, so much damage may occur to the ureter and kidney that the doctor may have to remove them. What would you call this operation?

_____ Neoureterocystostomy
_____ Obstructive uropathy
_____ Nephroureterectomy

6.24

Dr. Sharp identified a tumor growing on Mr. Carson Oma's ureter. He decided to remove the tumor. To remove the tumor Dr. Sharp cut out part of the ureter too. Next, Dr. Sharp sutured one end of the ureter to the other end. What is the name of this procedure?

_____ Neoureterocystostomy
_____ Ureteroureterostomy
_____ Ureterolysis

6.21

When urine, a watery substance, backs up in the kidneys, the kidneys swell up. This condition is called <u>hydronephrosis</u>. It is serious since it can kill cells in the kidneys.

Hydro- + *nephr-* + *-osis* describes this condition: *hydro-* = water or watery fluid; *nephr-* = kidney; *-osis* = disease

6.22

<u>Hydroureter</u> describes the condition where urine accumulates in the ureter.

If you break this big word, hydroureter, into its two smaller parts: *hydro-* + *-ureter*, you can more easily see the meaning: *hydro-* = water or watery fluid + *-ureter* = the tubes between the kidney and bladder.

6.23

<u>Nephroureterectomy</u> is the surgical removal of the kidney and the ureter.

Train your eye to break large words like this into smaller parts: *nephro-* = kidney + *ureter-* = ureter + *-ectomy* = surgical removal. Focus really hard on learning the roots and suffixes.

6.24

<u>Ureteroureterostomy</u> is the surgical joining of one part of the ureter to another part of the SAME ureter.

The word breaks down into *uretero-* + *uretero-* + *-stomy*. *-stomy* indicates the opening between the two parts of the ureter that are being joined. This operation is always performed on one and the same ureter.

Quick Review	
Ot- = ear	*-scope* = instrument used to examine
-scopy- = examining with an instrument	*-stomy* = a surgical opening

_____ 6.9 Uremia	**A.** Inflammation of the bladder
_____ 6.10 Proteinuria	**B.** Refers to the bladder
_____ 6.11 Cyst	**C.** Too much protein in the urine
_____ 6.12 Cystitis	**D.** A condition where the patient has too much urea in the blood.

6.25

There are lots of operations performed during which two body parts may be joined. There is a medical term that describes this procedure of joining two body parts. What is the term?

_____ Anastomosis   _____ Catheterization   _____ Lithotripsy

6.26

Which of the operations named below indicates that the ureter was joined to the intestine?

_____ Ureteroneocystostomy
_____ Ureteroenterostomy
_____ Ureteropyelostomy

6.27

Some operations are performed by inserting a surgical instrument through the urethra. What is the term for this type of operation?

_____ Aspiration procedures
_____ Urodynamic procedures
_____ Transurethral surgery

6.25

Anastomosis means to join two body parts.

If you look carefully at anaSTOMosis you'll notice that *stom-* (opening) is part of anaSTOMosis. Remember ureteroureteroSTOMY? In this type of operation, the doctor joins two body parts to recreate the opening. This type of operation is performed often: the ureter may be joined to itself, the other ureter, the intestine, the skin, or the bladder.

6.26

Ureteroenterostomy is the joining of the ureter and the intestine.

Uretero- refers to the ureter; *entero-* refers to the intestine and *-stomy* refers to the opening that is created by joining the two parts.

Take Note! Notice that sometimes *stom-* is used with operations that create artificial openings (colo-stomy) and sometimes with operations that repair a natural opening inside the body. How can you tell the difference? Usually, if the operation affects two body parts, both parts are included in the name of the operation. For example,

ureteroureterostomy – joins two parts of the same ureter
ureteroneocystostomy – joins the ureter and the bladder (*cyst-*)
ureterosigmoidostomy – joins the ureter and the sigmoid intestine.

Operations, that create an artificial opening to the skin surface, name only the body part where the opening is created. For example, ureterostomy – an opening created in the ureter (to drain urine from the body). Cystostomy – an opening created in the bladder (to drain urine from the body).

6.27

Transurethral surgery is surgery that goes through the urethra.

Transurethral surgery describes the path the doctor takes. The scope is pushed through (trans) the urethra to get to the bladder and the other organs.
Trans- = through + *-urethral* = urethra

Doctors often must perform an endoscopy to find and treat their patients' problems. They may use the endoscope to look into the bladder, the ureter, the pelvis or the prostate. Endoscopy is a general term that includes all these procedures. It gets its name from how these procedures are performed.

6.28

Dr. Sharp has a patient with a lesion in the bladder. He decides to use an endoscope to destroy the lesion. What is the name of this surgery?

CLUE

Find the word for bladder in the box at the beginning of the chapter.

_____ Cystourethroscopy   _____ Colonoscopy   _____ Anoscopy

6.29

When Dr. Sharp saw the lesion through the scope, he used fulguration (from the Greek for lightning flashes) to destroy the lesion tissue. What do you think fulguration is? A procedure that uses an instrument that destroys tissue by

_____ Freezing the tissue   _____ Using a laser beam
_____ Creating electric sparks that burn the tissue

6.30

Vesico- is a term that is also used to refer to the bladder. Which of these terms means incision into the bladder?

_____ Vesicocele   _____ Vesicotomy   _____ Vesicostomy

6.31

You've got this! Use your word power to figure out what this term means: Vesicoenteric. (*vesico- + enter- + -ic*)

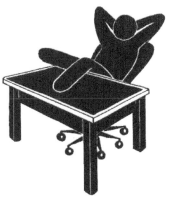

_____

6.28

Cystourethroscopy is an operation using an endoscope to treat a problem in the bladder, urethra, or any body part that can be reached through the bladder and the urethra.

Cystourethroscopy = *cysto-* (bladder) + *urethro-* (urethra) + *-scopy* (the technique of operating with a scope.)

6.29

Fulguration is creating electric sparks that burn the tissue.

Fulguration is one method of destroying lesions or undesirable tissue. This process uses an electric current to produce sparks to destroy the tissue.

6.30

Vesicotomy means an incision into the bladder.

Vesico- is from the Latin word for bladder. *-tomy* means incision. Therefore, vesicotomy is an incision into the bladder.

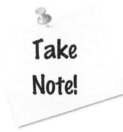

Take Note!

Don't' confuse *-tomy* (incision) with *-stomy* (surgical opening).

6.31

Vesicoenteric means pertaining to the bladder and the intestines.

Vesico- = bladder, *enter-* = intestines, and *-ic* = pertaining to.

Quick Review	
-lapaxy = to empty out	*Cyst-* = a pouch that contains liquid, bladder
-cele = swelling	*Hydro-* = water or watery fluid

Chapter Quiz 1 (Answers in Appendix A)

Choose the correct match.

_____ 6.1 X-raying the bladder and urethra	A. Urethrocystography
_____ 6.2 Endoscopy to crush stones in bladder	B. Transurethral
_____ 6.3 Infection of the triangular-shaped area at the bottom of the bladder	C. Ureterocele
_____ 6.4 Swelling of the wall of the ureter	D. Cystitis
_____ 6.5 Surgical fastening of the urethra to hold it in its normal position	E. Litholapaxy
_____ 6.6 Surgery that goes through the urethra	F. Catheterization
_____ 6.7 The process of inserting a tube into the bladder to withdraw urine	G. Trigonitis
_____ 6.8 Any procedure that joins two body parts	H. Fulguration
_____ 6.9 Destroying lesions with electric sparks	I. Urethropexy
_____ 6.10 Inflammation of the bladder	J. Anastomosis

You've got this! Use your new knowledge to decipher these words.

_____ 6.11 Cystorrhaphy	A. Surgical suture of the bladder
_____ 6.12 Cystoscopy	B. Procedure of x-raying the bladder
_____ 6.13 Cystoscope	C. X-ray of the bladder and the ureter
_____ 6.14 Cystography	D. Instrument for examining the bladder
_____ 6.15 Cystospasm	E. Examination of the bladder with a scope
_____ 6.16 Cystoureteritis	F. Involuntary contraction of the bladder
_____ 6.17 Cystourethritis	G. Inflammation of the ureter and the bladder
_____ 6.18 Cystoureterogram	H. Inflammation of the urethra and the bladder

Write-in the correct word from the list below.

6.19 Removing stones by cutting into the bladder _____

6.20 Infection of the urethra and trigone _____

6.21 Surgical removal of the bladder _____

6.22 Too much urea in the blood _____

6.23 Accumulation of urine in kidney _____

6.24 Condition where urine accumulates in the ureter _____

6.25 Too much protein in the urine _____

6.26 Long narrow tubes between the

        kidneys and the bladder _____

6.27 The canal from which we release

        urine from our bodies _____

6.28 Surgical cut into the bladder _____

Hydroureter	Hydronephrosis	Uremia
Cystectomy	Urethrotrigonitis	Cystolithotomy
Cystotomy	Urethra	Proteinuria
Ureter		

Chapter Quiz 2 (Answers in Appendix A)

Choose the correct match.

_____ 6.29 Transurethral	A. Too much urea in the blood
_____ 6.30 Cystolithotomy	B. X-raying the bladder and urethra
_____ 6.31 Catheterization	C. Removing stones by cutting into the bladder
_____ 6.32 Uremia	D. Surgical removal of the bladder
_____ 6.33 Cystectomy	E. Infection of the urethra and trigone
_____ 6.34 Urethrocystography	F. The process of inserting a tube into the bladder to withdraw urine
_____ 6.35 Urethrotrigonitis	G. Inflammation of the bladder
_____ 6.36 Hydronephrosis	H. Surgery that goes through the urethra
_____ 6.37 Trigonitis	I. Infection of the triangular-shaped area at the bottom of the bladder
_____ 6.38 Cystitis	J. Accumulation of urine in kidney

You've got this! Use your new knowledge to decipher these words.

_____ 6.39 Vesicosigmoidostomy	A. Concerning the bladder and the adbomen
_____ 6.40 Vesicoureteral	B. Incision into the neck of the bladder
_____ 6.41 Hydropericardium	C. Device for examining the urethra and bladder
_____ 6.42 Hydroma	D. X-raying the urethra and the bladder
_____ 6.43 Cystotrachelotomy	E. Concerning the bladder and the ureter
_____ 6.44 Cystourethroscope	F. Any cyst containing a watery substance
_____ 6.45 Cystourethrography	G. Surgical joining of the bladder and part of the colon
_____ 6.46 Vesicoabdominal	H. Accumulation of water in the pericardial sac

Write-in the correct word from the list below.

6.47 Using a scope to remove stones _____

6.48 Condition where urine accumulates in the ureter _____

6.49 Too much protein in the urine _____

6.50 Long narrow tubes between
        the kidneys and the bladder _____

6.51 Swelling of the wall of the ureter _____

6.52 Surgical cut into the bladder _____

6.53 Any procedure that joins two body parts _____

6.54 Surgical fastening of the urethra
        to hold it in its normal position _____

6.55 The canal from which we
        release urine from our bodies _____

6.56 Destroying lesions with electric sparks _____

Anastomosis	Litholapaxy	Ureterocele
Fulguration	Urethropexy	Cystotomy
Urethra	Ureter	Proteinuria
Hydroureter		

7

The Urinary System, Part 2: Are you kidney(ing) me?

Let's talk about a few more terms that relate to the urinary system.

It's all GREEK [or Latin] **to me!**

cystica – associated with cysts
diverticula – little sacs
fistula – abnormal opening
metro – measure
pyel – refers to pelvis of the kidney

7.1

Oscar Peabody has a kidney stone and Dr. Sharp is going to make a surgical incision into the pelvis of the kidney (the part of the kidney from which urine drains into the ureter). What is this procedure?

_____ Pyelotomy   _____ Pyelectomy   _____ Pyelostomy

7.2

One of Dr. Sharp's patients is scheduled for a pyelostomy. Dr. Sharp will

_____ Form a new kidney pelvis
_____ Create a surgical opening into the kidney pelvis
_____ Remove the kidney

7.3

Using your knowledge of word parts, when you want to refer to the skin and the kidney pelvis you would use the term:

_____ Subcutaneous   _____ Percutaneous   _____ Pyelocutaneous

7.1

<u>Pyelotomy</u> is a surgical incision into the pelvis of the kidney.

You have to put the word parts together. *Pyel-* is a word part that refers to the pelvis of the kidney. Remember, *-tomy* is the suffix that means cutting into a body part.

7.2

A pyelostomy is the <u>creation of a surgical opening into the kidney pelvis</u>.

Pyel- = pelvis of the kidney; *-stomy* = surgical opening into a body part.

7.3

<u>Pyelocutaneous</u> makes reference to the pelvis of the kidney and the skin.

Pyel- = pelvis of the kidney; *-cutaneous* = pertaining to the skin

 # Easily confused word parts

Don't be confused by similar word parts with different meanings!

-tomy – surgical incision **-stomy** – surgical opening **-ectomy** – surgical removal	**-graphy** – indicates a procedure **-graph** – the machine used to make an x-ray **-gram** – the written record
-osteo – bone **-oto** – ear	**stenosis** – narrowing **sclerosis** – hardening
myel – bone marrow **myo** – muscle	**arthro** – joint **athero** – fatty deposit
hypo – under, beneath, below **hyper** – over, above, excess	**pyelo** – pelvis of kidney **pylor** – refers to pylorus
derma – skin **-edema** - swelling	**-rrhage** – excessive flow or discharge **-rrhea** – indicates a discharge **-rrhaphy** – surgical suturing **-rrhexis** – rupture

7.4

Dr. Sharp has found it necessary to perform an ureteropyelostomy on a patient with a damaged urinary system. What will he do?

_____ Surgically create an opening into the ureter

_____ Remove a portion of the ureter and attach the cut end to a new opening in the kidney pelvis

_____ Surgically create an opening into the kidney

7.5

Challenge your inquiring mind: Dr. Sharp is monitoring Suzie Belle's condition. He has requested ureteropyelography. He requested

_____ The graphical report from the x-ray examination of the ureter

_____ The machine used to perform an x-ray examination of the kidney

_____ The x-ray examination of the ureter and kidney pelvis after injection of a dye

7.6

You're on a roll! Let's go for another. Which of the following is the word for inflammation of the kidney pelvis and the ureter associated with small cysts?

_____ Pyelitis

_____ Ureteropyelonephritis

_____ Pyeloureteritis cystica

7.7

Now let's broaden our vocabulary a little more. Diverticula are little sacs or pouches in an organ such as the intestines. If a patient has diverticulitis, what do you think the person has?

_____ A diverted ureter

_____ Little inflamed sacs in the intestines

_____ Little sacs in the intestines have become hard

7.4
Ureteropyelostomy is the <u>removal of a portion of the ureter and attachment of the cut end to a new opening in the kidney pelvis.</u>

Uretero- = ureter; *pyel-* = kidney pelvis; *-stomy-* = surgical opening into a body part

7.5
Ureteropyelography is <u>the x-ray examination of the ureter and kidney pelvis after the injection of a dye.</u>

Uretero- = ureter; *pyel-* = kidney pelvis; *-graphy* = process of making a record

7.6
<u>Pyeloureteritis cystica</u> is the inflammation of the kidney pelvis and the ureter associated with small cysts.

Pyel- = kidney pelvis; *ureter-* = ureter; *-itis* = inflammation; *cystica* = associated with cysts

7.7
Diverticulitis is <u>the inflammation of diverticula (little sacs) in the intestines.</u>

Diverticula- = little sacs; *-itis* = inflammation

QUICK QUIZ *(Answers in Appendix A)*

_____ 7.1 *Hydro-*   *A.* Vein

_____ 7.2 *Vesico-*   *B.* Water or watery like substance

_____ 7.3 *Lipo-*   *C.* Fat tissue

_____ 7.4 *Phlebo-*   *D.* The bladder

7.8

The little swollen sacs don't have to be in the intestinal tract. Sally is bothered by a urethral diverticulum. She suffers from

_____ A twisted urethra

_____ A swollen sac in the ureteral wall

_____ A swollen sac in the wall of the urethra

7.9

Patsy has been experiencing urinary problems. Dr. Sharp is checking the cystogram, which was obtained from a procedure called cystography. Cystography is

_____ Physical examination of the bladder

_____ X-ray examination of the kidney

_____ X-ray examination of the bladder after the injection of dye

7.10

Dr. Sharp wants a to see a visual image of the pressure in Luke's bladder at various stages as it fills with urine. He wants a

_____ Cystometrogram

_____ Cystometer

_____ Cystography

CLUE

You learned this key suffix in the very first chapter, page 6!

7.11

You're already familiar with the word parts *cyst-* and *vesico-*. What is a vesicouterine fistula?

_____ An abnormal opening between the bladder and the ureter

_____ An abnormal opening between the uterus and the bladder

_____ An abnormal opening between the kidney and the ureter

7.8

A urethral diverticulum is <u>a swollen sac in the wall of the urethra</u>.

Urethral = pertaining to the urethra; diverticulum = swollen sac

7.9

Cystography is the <u>x-ray examination of the bladder after the injection of a dye</u>.

Cysto- = bladder; *-graphy* = process of making a record

7.10

Dr. Sharp wants a cystometrogram, a record of the pressure in the bladder at various stages as it fills with urine.

Cysto- = bladder; *metro-* = measure; *-gram* = record

7.11

A vesicouterine fistula is <u>an opening between the uterus and the bladder</u>.

Vesico- = bladder; *-uterine* = uterus; *fistula* = abnormal opening

---

QUICK QUIZ *(Answers in Appendix A)*

_____ 7.5 Trigonitis

A. A small tube used to open up a closed body channel or to maintain an opening in a body channel

_____ 7.6 Urethrotrigonitis

B. Fixing or fastening the urethra to the wall of the vagina with sutures

_____ 7.7 Catheterization

C. Inflammation of the trigone

_____ 7.8 Urethropexy

D. Infection of the urethra and the trigone

And, here's a few more
terms for this chapter.

It's all GREEK [or Latin] **to me!**

-genic – producing, arising from
meato – a passage or opening
renal – refers to the kidney
resection – removal of a section

7.12

A vesicocutaneous fistula would involve the

_____ Kidney and skin   _____ Liver and skin   _____ Bladder and skin

7.13

And, of course, a fistula involving
the kidney and the skin would be:

_____ Cystocutaneous
_____ Gastrocutaneous
_____ Nephrocutaneous

CLUE

You know that the suffix,
-cutaneous refers to the
skin, so pay attention to
the prefix!

7.14

You've got this! Dr. Sharp has found it
necessary to perform a vesicostomy on a new
patient. What is a vesicostomy?
(*vesico-* + *-stomy*)

_____

7.15

It may be necessary for Dr. Sharp to surgically stabilize Sandy's bladder and
urethra. This procedure is called

_____ Vesicostomy   _____ Vesicourethropexy   _____ Urethrography

7.12

A vesicocutaneous fistula would involve the <u>bladder and the skin</u>.

Vesico- = bladder; *-cutaneous* = pertaining to the skin; fistula = abnormal opening

7.13

<u>Nephrocutaneous</u> denotes an association with the kidney and the skin.

Nephro- = kidney; *-cutaneous* = pertaining to the skin

Take Note!

You know that *nephro-* refers to the kidney. That's easy enough. Oh, but wait. There's another term that refers to the kidney, **renal**. A patient is suffering from hardening of the arteries of the kidney. Would you refer to this as renal sclerosis or nephrosclerosis? Well, both are correct, actually. *Renal* comes from Latin while *nephro* comes from Greek.

7.14

When Dr. Sharp performs the vesicostomy, he will <u>surgically create an opening into the bladder</u>.

Vesico- = bladder; *-stomy* = surgical opening into a body part

7.15

<u>Vesicourethropexy</u> is the surgical fixation of the bladder and urethra.

Vesico- means bladder; *urethro-* pertains to the urethra; *-pexy* means fixation.

Quick Review	
-pepsia- = digestion	*Trans-* = through
Meno- = indicates menstruation	*Mega-* = large

7.16

Sometimes Dr. Sharp finds it necessary to remove a portion of a body part that is diseased or damaged. This procedure is called

_____ Redirection   _____ Resection   _____ Incision

7.17

A transurethral surgical procedure is performed through the:

_____ ureter   _____ urethra   _____ kidney

7.18

Sometimes transurethral surgery involves a meatotomy to enlarge the external urethral opening. In performing the procedure, Dr. Sharp will

_____ Remove the urethra   _____ Repair the urethra
_____ Make an incision into the urethral meatus to enlarge the opening

7.19

Some of the conditions Dr. Sharp encounters are nephrogenic. Such conditions are produced by/arising from the:

_____ Bladder   _____ Kidney   _____ Ureter

7.20

Nephrogenic diabetes, then is a form of diabetes caused by a malfunction of the

_____ Kidney   _____ Pancreas   _____ Liver

7.21

You've got this! Use your word power to figure out what this medical term means: Nephrography. (*nephro-* + *-graphy*)

_____

7.16

Resection is the surgical removal of a section of any part of the body.

The physician performs a resection if s/he removes a part of the bladder, a part of a bone, or a part of any body organ or structure. Resection is sometimes performed as transurethral surgery.

7.17

Transurethral surgery is performed through the urethra.

Trans- = through; *-urethral* = pertaining to the urethra

7.18

A meatotomy is an incision into the urinary meatus to enlarge the external urethral opening.

Meato- = a passage or opening (e.g., the opening into the urethra); *-tomy* = surgical cut into a body part

7.19

Nephrogenic means arising from the kidney.

The suffix *-genic* indicates generation or production. *Nephro-* = pertaining to the kidneys. Put them together and you have nephrogenic, coming from or arising from the kidney.

7.20

Nephrogenic diabetes is caused by a malfunction of the kidney.

7.21

Nephrography is taking an x-ray of the kidney.

Nephro- refers to the kidney and *-graphy* is the act of taking an x-ray.

Chapter Quiz 1 (Answers in Appendix A)

Choose the correct match.

_____ 7.1 Incision into kidney pelvis	A. Pyeloureteritis cystica
_____ 7.2 Refers to kidney pelvis and skin	B. Ureteropyelostomy
_____ 7.3 Create a surgical opening into the pelvis of the kidney	C. Vesicouterine fistula
_____ 7.4 X-raying bladder after injecting dye	D. Resection
_____ 7.5 Remove a portion of the ureter and attach cut end to opening in the kidney pelvis	E. Pyelotomy
_____ 7.6 Inflammation of kidney pelvis and ureter with small cysts	F. Pyelocutaneous
_____ 7.7 A record of pressure in a bladder	G. Diverticulitis
_____ 7.8 Partial removal of a body organ or structure	H. Cystometrogram
_____ 7.9 Abnormal opening between uterus and the bladder	I. Pyelostomy
_____ 7.10 The inflammation of little swollen sacs in the intestines	J. Cystography

You've got this! Use your new knowledge to decipher these words.

_____ 7.11 Pyelitis	A. Originating in the heart
_____ 7.12 Pyelopathy	B. Any disease of the pelvis of the kidney
_____ 7.13 Pyelocystitis	C. Inflammation of the kidney pelvis
_____ 7.14 Pyelonephritis	D. Inflammation of the liver and kidney
_____ 7.15 Cardiorenal	E. Inflammation of the renal pelvis and bladder
_____ 7.16 Cardiogenic	F. Having its origin in the liver
_____ 7.17 Hepatogenic	G. Pertaining to the heart and kidney
_____ 7.18 Hepatonephritis	H. Inflammation of the kidney pelvis and the kidney

Write-in the correct word from the list below.

7.19 Involving kidney and the skin _____

7.20 Surgery performed through the urethra _____

7.21 Arising from the kidney _____

7.22 Hardening of arteries of the kidney _____

7.23 A swollen sac in the wall of the urethra _____

7.24 An incision into the urinary meatus _____

7.25 The surgical fixation of the bladder and urethra _____

7.26 Surgically create opening into bladder _____

7.27 X-ray examination of the ureter and kidney pelvis _____

7.28 Concerning the bladder and the skin _____

Transurethral	Meatotomy	Vesicostomy
Ureteropyelography	Nephrogenic	Renal sclerosis
Vesicocutaneous	Vesicourethropexy	Nephrocutaneous
Urethral diverticulum		

Chapter Quiz 2 (Answers in Appendix A)

Choose the correct match.

_____ 7.29 Transurethral	A. The surgical fixation of the bladder and urethra
_____ 7.30 Renal sclerosis	B. An incision into the urinary meatus
_____ 7.31 Nephrocutaneous	C. Surgically create an opening into the bladder
_____ 7.32 Nephrogenic	D. A swollen sac in the wall of the urethra
_____ 7.33 Vesicourethropexy	E. X-ray examination of the ureter and kidney pelvis
_____ 7.34 Meatotomy	F. Surgery performed through the urethra
_____ 7.35 Urethral diverticulum	G. Concerning the bladder and the skin
_____ 7.36 Vesicostomy	H. Hardening of arteries of the kidney
_____ 7.37 Ureteropyelography	I. Arising from the kidney
_____ 7.38 Vesicocutaneous	J. Involving kidney and the skin

You've got this! Use your new knowledge to decipher these words.

_____ 7.39 Gastrogenic	A. Originating in the stomach
_____ 7.40 Bronchogenic	B. Renal hernia or swelling
_____ 7.41 Otogenic	C. Surgical fixation of the kidney
_____ 7.42 Rhinogenic	D. Surgery to repair the pelvis of the kidney
_____ 7.43 Pyeloplasty	E. Originating in the windpipe
_____ 7.44 Nephrocele	F. Enlarged kidney
_____ 7.45 Nephromegaly	G. Originating in the ear
_____ 7.46 Nephropexy	H. Originating in the nose

Write-in the correct word from the list below.

7.47 A record of pressure in a bladder _____

7.48 X-raying bladder after injecting dye _____

7.49 Remove a portion of ureter and attach
       cut end to opening in kidney pelvis _____

7.50 Create a surgical opening
       into the pelvis of the kidney _____

7.51 Incision into kidney pelvis _____

7.52 Inflammation of kidney pelvis
       and ureter associated with small cysts _____

7.53 Abnormal opening between uterus and the bladder _____

7.54 Partial removal of a body organ or structure _____

7.55 The inflammation of little
       swollen sacs in the intestines _____

7.56 Refers to kidney pelvis and skin _____

Ureteropyelostomy	Resection	Pyelotomy
Pyeloureteritis cystica	Pyelostomy	Vesicouterine fistula
Cystography	Pyelocutaneous	Cystometrogram
Diverticulitis		

8

The Cardiovascular System:
The heart of the matter

Let's look at a few Latin and Greek terms that are used when describing diseases and treatment for the cardiovascular system.

> **It's all GREEK** [or Latin] **to me!**
>
> **brady** – slow
> **defibrillator** – stops chaotic heartbeat
> **tachy** – swift, fast
> **vasculo** – refers to the blood vessels

8.1

What about this word: cardiovascular? What is the cardiovascular system?

_____ Heart & valves   _____ Heart & blood vessels   _____ Heart & lungs

8.2

Remember that *peri-* means near? What is the pericardium?

_____ The valves within   _____ The sac enclosing   _____ The cells that
    the heart   the heart   initiate the
                                   heartbeat

8.3

A person comes to the doctor complaining of fever, dry cough, upset stomach, and irregular heartbeat. The doctor diagnoses the problem as pericarditis. How would you describe the patient's condition?

_____ The arteries near the heart are inflamed
_____ The pericardium is inflamed
_____ The muscles near the heart are infected

8.1

Cardiovascular refers to the <u>heart & blood</u> <u>vessels</u>.

Vasculo- is from a Latin word, meaning "small vessel." When you put *cardio-* with *-vascular*, you are referring to the heart and the blood vessels, the cardiovascular system.

8.2

The pericardium is <u>the sac enclosing the</u> <u>heart</u>.

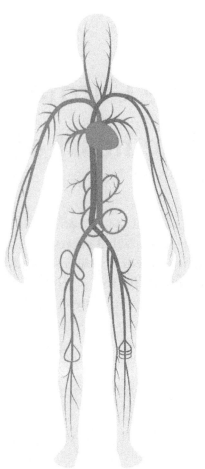

Remember, *cardi-* means heart and *peri-* means surrounding.

8.3

Pericarditis is an <u>inflammation of the</u> <u>pericardium</u>.

Pericarditis is *pericard- + -itis*. *Pericard-* refers to the pericardium and *-itis* is a suffix meaning inflamed.

Quick Review	
Vesico- = refers to the bladder	*-pexy* = hold or fasten
-rrhage = abnormal or excessive flow	*-rrhaphy* = surgical suturing
-genic = produced by or arising from	*-spasm* = the involuntary contraction of a muscle

8.4

Dr. Sharp created an opening in the pericardium to drain the fluid from the inflamed pericardium. What did Dr. Sharp do?

_____ A pericardiorrhaphy   _____ A pericardiopexy
_____ A pericardiostomy

8.5

The infection in the pericardium refuses to heal. Finally Dr. Sharp removes the infected area of the pericardium. What procedure did Dr. Sharp perform?

_____ Pericardiotomy

_____ Pericardiocentesis

_____ Pericardiectomy

CLUE These are some common suffixes that are easily confused, so it's good to memorize them!

8.6

While Dr. Sharp performed the procedure, the patient was on the heart/lung machine to move the blood around the heart. What is the name for using the heart/lung machine?

_____ Cardiopulmonary bypass   _____ Cardiotachometer
_____ Cardiopneumograph

8.7

Later that day, Dr. Sharp saw a patient. Both his pericardium and the muscular wall of his heart were inflamed.What condition describes this patient?

_____ Pericarditis   _____ Myopericarditis   _____ Pleuropericarditis

8.8

Dr. Sharp sees a patient whose heart rate is over 100 beats per minute. That's too fast. What's the name of this condition?

_____ Pericardial effusion   _____ Tachycardia   _____ Mitral stenosis

8.4

A <u>pericardiostomy</u> is an opening in the pericardium.

Pericardiostomy is made up of *pericardio-* + *-stomy*. *-stomy* is from a Greek word meaning mouth. A mouth is an opening!

8.5

A <u>pericardiectomy</u> is the removal of all or part of the pericardium.

These are some common suffixes: *-ectomy* is a suffix meaning surgical removal or excision. *-tomy* is a surgical incision; *-stomy* is a surgical opening.

8.6

Using the <u>cardiopulmonary bypass</u> machine, the blood literally goes around or bypasses the heart.

Cardio- + *-pulmonary* = heart plus lungs. Bypass means to go around.

8.7

<u>Myopericarditis</u> is an inflammation of the muscular wall of the heart and the pericardium.

Myo- means muscles; *pericard-* stands for pericardium; *-itis* means inflammation.

8.8

<u>Tachycardia</u> is the abnormal rapidity of heart action.

Tachy- is a Greek word, meaning swift and *–cardia* refers to the heart.

Here's a few more terms associated with the cardiovascular system.

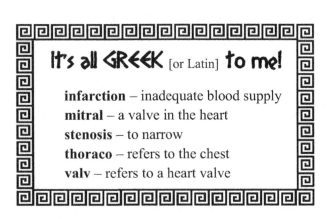

It's all GREEK [or Latin] to me!

infarction – inadequate blood supply
mitral – a valve in the heart
stenosis – to narrow
thoraco – refers to the chest
valv – refers to a heart valve

8.9

Dr. Sharp sees a patient in the emergency room with an irregular fast heartbeat, which may cause cardiac arrest. To treat the condition, Dr. Sharp uses an electrical device that applies countershocks to the heart. What is the name of this device?

_____ Defibrillator   _____ Cardionector   _____ Cardiogram

8.10

Dr. Sharp sees a new patient. She has a really slow heartbeat, less than 60 beats per minute. What is the name of this condition?

_____ Mitral insufficiency   _____ Hypoplasia   _____ Bradycardia

8.11

Dr. Sharp implants a permanent pacemaker to regulate his patient's heartbeat. To insert it, he makes an incision into the chest. What is the name for this incision?

_____ Mammotomy   _____ Arthrotomy   _____ Thoracotomy

8.12

Dr. Sharp sees a new patient who has had a heart attack because of damage to the heart muscle. What is the medical term for this condition?

_____ Cerebral embolism   _____ Ventricular   _____ Myocardial
                                    tachycardia   infarction

8.13

Dr. Sharp sees a new patient. She has a problem with one of her heart valves. The opening in the valve has narrowed, due to scarring from rheumatic fever. What is the name of this condition?

_____ Valvulitis   _____ Cardiomegaly   _____ Mitral stenosis

8.9

A <u>defibrillator</u> stops fibrillation, a heartbeat that is chaotic.

It is an electrical device that applies countershocks to the heart with the hope that this will allow the heart's normal pacemaker to take over.

8.10

<u>Bradycardia</u> is a slow heartbeat, usually one under 60 beats in adults. *Brady-* is a Greek word meaning slow.

8.11

<u>Thoracotomy</u> is a surgical incision into the chest.

Thorax is the Greek word for chest. *Thoraco-* refers to chest; *-tomy* is a suffix meaning surgical incision.

8.12

<u>Myocardial infarction</u> is a term for heart attack.

Infarction describes a condition where an area of muscle tissue is damaged or dies because it does not receive enough blood. *Myo-* indicates muscle and *cardial* indicates heart.

8.13

<u>Mitral stenosis</u> is the narrowing of a heart valve.

Mitral is the name of the valve between the right atrium and the right ventricle of the heart. Stenosis is from Greek, meaning the act of narrowing.

Quick Review	
-graph = an instrument used to record something	*-graphy* = the procedure used to record something
Pyelo- = the pelvis of the kidney	*Renal* = refers to the kidney
Duodeno- = portion of the small intestine	*Uria-* = refers to urinary tract

8.14

Dr. Sharp makes a surgical incision into the valve. What is the name of this procedure?

_____ Valvectomy

_____ Valvulitis

_____ Valvotomy

CLUE

Concentrate on the suffix! It's one of those easily confused words described on page 116.

8.15

Dr. Sharp sees a patient whose valve fails to close, allowing the blood to flow back into the heart chamber. What is the name of this condition?

_____ Valvulitis   _____ Mitral stenosis   _____ Mitral insufficiency

8.16

Dr. Sharp repairs the valve, rather than replacing it. What is the name of this procedure?

_____ Valvectomy

_____ Valvotomy

_____ Valvuloplasty

CLUE

Look at the suffix! Dr. Sharp is <u>repairing</u> the valve!

8.17

Dr. Sharp sees a child with a congenital heart problem. He has a lesion in the wall between the atrium and ventricle. To repair the condition, Dr. Sharp closes the opening in the wall. What is the name of this condition?

_____ Atrial septal defect   _____ Coronary arterial fistula   _____ Cardiac arrest

Quick Review	
Procto- = anus	*-itis* = inflammation
-ectomy = surgical excision	*-tomy* = a surgical cut

8.14

A <u>valvotomy</u> is a surgical incision into the valve.

Don't forget! *-tomy* is a suffix meaning surgical incision. *Valv-* refers to the heart valve.

8.15

<u>Mitral insufficiency</u> is when the valve fails to close.

8.16

<u>Valvuloplasty</u> is a procedure to form, mold, repair, or reconstruct the damaged valve.

Valv- refers to the heart valve and *-plasty* is from a Greek word, meaning to form.

8.17

<u>Atrial septal defect</u> is a defect between the atrium and ventricle.

Atrial is the adjective form of the name of the heart chamber, atrium. Septal is the adjective form of the name of the wall, septum, between the atrium and the ventricle.

Sometimes when a fetus is growing, problems arise because the structure, position, or form of an organ does not develop normally. This is called an anomaly.

When this happens in the heart, it is very dangerous because the baby cannot get oxygenated blood to the body. Often the doctors will have to operate immediately upon delivery.

Quick Review	
Metr- = uterus	*Cephal-* = head
-plasty = surgical repair or reconstruction	*-scler* = hard

QUICK QUIZ (Answers in Appendix A)

_____ 8.1 Vesicostomy

_____ 8.2 Pyelotomy

_____ 8.3 Pyelostomy

_____ 8.4 Cystography

A. The x-ray examination of the bladder

B. Surgical incision into the pelvis of the kidney

C. The creation of a surgical opening into the kidney pelvis

D. Surgically create an opening into the bladder

8.18

The patient's aortic valve is narrowing. What is this condition called?

_____ Aortic stenosis   _____ Aortosclerosis   _____ Aortalgia

8.19

Someone who has hardening of the aorta has a condition called:

_____ Aortic stenosis   _____ Aortosclerosis   _____ Aortalgia

8.20

To establish an adequate mix of oxygenated and unoxygenated blood, Dr. Sharp created an opening in the wall of the atrium. What is the name of this procedure?

_____ Atrial septectomy   _____ Atrial septotomy   _____ Atrial septostomy

8.21

You've got this! Here's a medical term we haven't shown you yet, but you'll be able to decipher its meaning. What does pneumopericardium mean?
(*pneumo-* + *-pericardium*)

_____

8.18

Narrowing of the aortic valve is called <u>aortic stenosis</u>.

Stenosis means narrowing.

8.19

<u>Aortosclerosis</u> is hardening of the aorta.

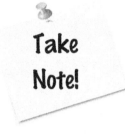

Aorto- refers to the aorta and *-sclerosis* means hardening.

They look similar, but notice the difference between **stenosis** *and* **sclerosis**

8.20

<u>Atrial septostomy</u> is the surgical creation of an opening, in this case to allow the oxygenated and unoxygenated blood to mix.

Remember *–stomy*? It is from a Greek word meaning mouth - an opening.

8.21

Pneumopericardium is <u>air or gas in the pericardial sac</u>.

Pneumopericardium is a big word but easy enough to break down: *pneumo-* stands for air and *-pericardium* refers to the pericardium (the sac surrounding the heart).

QUICK QUIZ *(Answers in Appendix A)*

_____ 8.5 Cardiopulmonary bypass	**A.** An abnormally fast heart rate
_____ 8.6 Pericardiectomy	**B.** A slow heartbeat
_____ 8.7 Tachycardia	**C.** When a patient is on the heart/lung machine
_____ 8.8 Bradycardia	**D.** The removal of all or part of the pericardium

---

Chapter Quiz 1 (Answers in Appendix A)

Choose the correct match.

_____ 8.1 Device that stops arrhythmic heartbeats	A. Pericardiectomy
_____ 8.2 Air or gas in the pericardial sac	B. Pneumopericardium
_____ 8.3 Inflammation of the heart	C. Anomaly
_____ 8.4 Hardening of the aorta	D. Thoracotomy
_____ 8.5 Inflamed heart muscles and pericardium	E. Vascular
_____ 8.6 Excision of the pericardium	F. Carditis
_____ 8.7 A heartbeat that is too slow	G. Aortosclerosis
_____ 8.8 A surgical incision into the chest	H. Defibrillator
_____ 8.9 An abnormal structure, form or position	I. Bradycardia
_____ 8.10 Refers to the blood vessels	J. Myopericarditis

You've got this! Use your new knowledge to decipher these words.

_____ 8.11 Bradyuria	A. Instrument for the inspection of the chest cavity
_____ 8.12 Tachygastria	B. Incision through the chest into the bronchus
_____ 8.13 Thoracopathy	C. Reconstruction of the chest and lung
_____ 8.14 Thoracoplasty	D. Diagnostic examination of the chest cavity using a scope
8.15 Thoracopneumoplasty	E. Slowness in passing urine
_____ 8.16 Thoracobronchotomy	F. Reconstruction of the chest
_____ 8.17 Thoracoscope	G. A disease of the chest
_____ 8.18 Thoracoscopy	H. Increased rate of contractions of the stomach

Write-in the correct word from the list below.

8.19 A valve that fails to close _____

8.20 Surgical repair of a valve _____

8.21 A heartbeat that is too fast _____

8.22 A valve whose opening is too narrow _____

8.23 Surgical opening into a heart wall _____

8.24 Surgical incision into a heart valve _____

8.25 Procedure using heart/lung machine _____

8.26 Inflamed pericardium _____

8.27 Refers to the heart and blood vessels _____

8.28 The sac surrounding the heart _____

Valvuloplasty	Cardiopulmonary bypass	Mitral insufficiency
Mitral stenosis	Pericardium	Tachycardia
Cardiovascular	Septostomy	Valvotomy
Pericarditis		

Chapter Quiz 2 (Answers in Appendix A)

Choose the correct match.

_____ 8.29 Valvuloplasty	A. Cardiovascular
_____ 8.30 Mitral stenosis	B. Procedure using heart/lung machine
_____ 8.31 Valvotomy	C. Surgical incision into a heart valve
_____ 8.32 Pericarditis	D. Surgical opening into a heart wall
_____ 8.33 Mitral insufficiency	E. A heartbeat that is too fast
_____ 8.34 Tachycardia	F. A valve whose opening is too narrow
_____ 8.35 Septostomy	G. A valve that fails to close
_____ 8.36 Cardiopulmonary bypass	H. Inflamed pericardium
_____ 8.37 Pericardium	I. The sac surrounding the heart
_____ 8.38 Refers to the heart and blood vessels	J. Surgical repair of a valve

You've got this! Use your new knowledge to decipher these words.

_____ 8.39 Bradypnea	A. Narrowness of the chest area
_____ 8.40 Thoracostenosis	B. Increased heart rate alternating with slow rate
_____ 8.41 Proctostenosis	C. Narrowing of the bronchial tubes
_____ 8.42 Bradytachycardia	D. Narrowing of the intestines
_____ 8.43 Bronchostenosis	E. Narrowing of the nasal passage
_____ 8.44 Blepharostenosis	F. Abnormally slow breathing
_____ 8.45 Rhinostenosis	G. Unable to open the eye normally
_____ 8.46 Enterostenosis	H. Narrowing of the anus

Write-in the correct word from the list below.

8.47 Device that stops arrhythmic heartbeats _____

8.48 Hardening of the aorta _____

8.49 Excision of the pericardium _____

8.50 Air or gas in the pericardial sac _____

8.51 An abnormal structure, form or position _____

8.52 Refers to the blood vessels _____

8.53 Inflamed heart muscles and pericardium _____

8.54 Inflammation of the heart _____

8.55 A surgical incision into the chest _____

8.56 A heartbeat that is too slow _____

Vascular	Anomaly	Defibrillator
Thoracotomy	Aortosclerosis	Pericardiectomy
Bradycardia	Myopericarditis	Pneumopericardium
Carditis		

9

The Vascular System: Veins inside and out

In the last lesson, you learned some basic words used when describing diseases of and treatment for the cardiovascular system. The last lesson focused on the

> **It's all GREEK** [or Latin] **to me!**
>
> **athero** – fatty deposit
> **lumen** – space within a blood vessel
> **thrombo** – refers to a blood clot

heart. This lesson we'll focus on terms used with the vascular system, the arteries and veins.

9.1

The aorta is the main trunk of the arterial system of the body, the artery that has its origin in the left ventricle of the heart. The patient's aorta is inflamed. What is the name of this condition?

_____ Aortoplasty   _____ Aortitis   _____ Aortotomy

9.2

An infant is born with a fibromuscular ridge growing inside the space of the aorta. This growth is narrowing the space inside the vessel, restricting the blood flow. What is the name of this condition?

_____ Aortic stenosis   _____ Aortic annulus   _____ Aortic suspension

9.3

What is the name of the space within the aorta through which blood flows?

_____ Intima   _____ Tunica media   _____ Lumen

9.1

<u>Aortitis</u> is inflammation of the aorta.

-itis means inflammation. The aorta carries oxygenated blood from the heart to all the limbs and organs (except the lungs) of the body.

9.2

<u>Aortic stenosis</u> is the narrowing of the passage through which the blood flows in the aorta.

Stenosis means the constriction or narrowing of a passage or orifice.

9.3

The space within the aorta through which blood flows is the <u>lumen</u>.

Lumen is the space within an artery, the intestines or a tube. It comes from the Latin for 'an opening'.

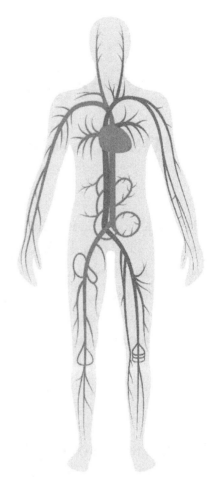

Here's a few more medical terms to take a look at.

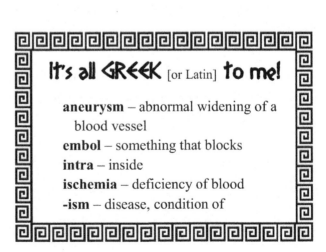

It's all GREEK [or Latin] to me!

aneurysm – abnormal widening of a blood vessel
embol – something that blocks
intra – inside
ischemia – deficiency of blood
-ism – disease, condition of

9.4

A patient comes to Dr. Sharp with narrowed arteries because of fatty degeneration or thickening of the walls. What do you call this condition?

_____ Thrombolysis _____ Apheresis _____ Atherosclerosis

9.5

Dr. Sharp performed a procedure to widen the inner space of the artery and remove the plaque from the artery wall. What did Dr. Sharp do?

_____ Transluminal atherectomy _____ Thromboendarterectomy _____ Embolectomy

9.6

Dr. Sharp sees a patient who has a blood clot developing. What is the name of this condition?

CLUE

See the Greek/Latin box on the facing page!

_____ Aortic stenosis _____ Thrombosis _____ Aneurysm

9.7

Dr. Sharp gave the patient medicine to thin the blood clot. However, it loosened and was carried through the blood stream until, at a smaller arterial branch, it blocked the blood flow. What is the name of this condition?

_____ Embolism _____ Aortitis _____ Aortic stenosis

9.8

Later that day, Dr. Sharp saw a patient. Tests showed that he had a weak spot on the subclavian artery, where the wall had thinned and stretched, widening the vessel. What is the name of this condition?

_____ Aortic stenosis _____ Atherosclerosis _____ Aneurysm

9.4

Atherosclerosis is the most common form of hardening of the arteries.

Athero- is from the Greek word meaning porridge, a thick soup. *-sclerosis* is from the Greek word to harden. The lumen becomes narrower and the walls of the arteries lose their elasticity.

9.5

Transluminal atherectomy is a procedure to remove plaque from the arterial wall.

Trans- + *-luminal* means through the inner space (lumen). *Ather-* + *-ectomy* means the surgical removal of the thickness of plaque.

9.6

Thrombosis is the formation, development or existence of a blood clot.

Thromb- refers to a blood clot and *–osis* means condition of.

9.7

An embolism is when a vessel is blocked.

Embol- is from a Greek word, meaning stopper. *–ism*, like *-osis*, means disease or condition of. Embolism literally means a vessel is blocked or stopped up.

9.8

An aneurysm is an abnormal widening of a blood vessel due to a congenital problem or a weakness of the vessel wall.

It comes from a Greek word meaning widening.

QUICK QUIZ (Answers in Appendix A)	
_____ 9.1 *Tachy-*	*A.* Slow
_____ 9.2 *Brady-*	*B.* Surrounding
_____ 9.3 *Peri-*	*C.* Muscle
_____ 9.4 *Myo-*	*D.* Fast

9.9

Dr. Sharp removes a blood clot from the site on the aortoiliac artery where the clot was forming. What's the name of this procedure?

_____ Thrombectomy   _____ Embolectomy   _____ Endarterectomy

9.10

Dr. Sharp removes a blood clot that has broken loose from its original site and is now blocking an artery. What is the name of this procedure?

_____ Thrombectomy   _____ Embolectomy   _____ Thromboendarterectomy

9.11

Dr. Sharp removes a blood clot and the inner wall of the artery, which has become infected. What is the name of this procedure?

_____ Thrombectomy   _____ Embolectomy   _____ Thromboendarterectomy

9.12

Dr. Sharp sees a new patient whose femoral vein is inflamed, as a result of a forming blood clot. What's the name
of this condition?

_____ Thrombolysis

_____ Thrombophlebitis

_____ Varicose veins

CLUE

Your clues are: blood clot, vein and inflamed.

9.13

Dr. Sharp sees a new patient. She has an abnormal opening that is joining one of her arteries with a vein. What do you call this condition?

_____ Stenosis   _____ Hypotension   _____ Fistula

9.9

Thrombectomy is the surgical removal of a blood clot.

Thromb- comes from thrombus, meaning blood clot and *–ectomy* refers to the surgical removal of something.

9.10

An embolectomy is the surgical removal of an embolus, any material that is blocking a blood vessel.

Embolectomy is made up of two word parts: *embol-* refers to embolism and *–ectomy*, to remove.

9.11

Thromboendarterectomy is the removal of a blood clot and the inner wall of an artery.

Thromboendarterectomy is a huge word, made up of smaller words. *Thrombo-* means blood clot; *end-* means inner; *arter-* means artery; *-ectomy* means surgical removal.

9.12

Thrombophlebitis is the condition of a vein becoming inflamed as the result of a blood clot.

Thrombophlebitis is made up of 3 important word parts: *thrombo-* meaning blood clot; *phleb-* meaning vein; *-itis* meaning inflammation.

9.13

A fistula is an abnormal joining of one vessel to another.

Fistula is from a Latin word meaning pipe. Like a pipe, it is a tubelike passage from a normal vessel to another. A fistula may be caused by a congenital problem, an injury or an inflammatory process.

9.14

Dr. Sharp sees a new patient. Her arteries have narrowed to the point where she is getting dizzy. Dr. Sharp performs an operation where he widens the artery by passing a balloon through the space within the artery. What's this procedure's name?

_____ Transluminal   _____ Aortoplasty   _____ Transcatheter
     angioplasty   therapy

9.15

Dr. Sharp performs angioplasty on a blood vessel in the chest. How would you describe this procedure?

_____ Intra-abdominal   _____ Intrathoracic   _____ Percutaneous

9.16

Because of a congenital problem, an infant must have his aorta reconstructed. What is the name of this procedure?

_____ Aortoplasty
_____ Aortopexy
_____ Aortic reconstructus

CLUE

We learned the suffix for reconstruction on page 29!

9.17

Dr. Sharp sees a patient whose blood vessels in her hip region are becoming too narrow to support the surrounding tissue. What is the name of this condition?

_____ Phlebostenosis   _____ Myocardial ischemia   _____ Angiostenosis

9.14

Transluminal angioplasty is widening an artery by passing a balloon through the space within the artery.

Transluminal, means through the inner space of the vessel. Angioplasty is the repair of a blood vessel. In this case, the doctor widened it.

9.15

Intrathoracic means inside the chest.

Another word for chest is thorax. The adjective form of thorax is thoracic. Inside the chest is intrathoracic. *Intra-* = inside and *–thoracic* = chest.

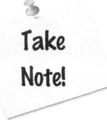

Take Note!

Sometimes several medical terms will have the same meaning.
Intra- and *endo-* both mean inside.

9.16

Aortoplasty is the reconstruction or repair of the aorta.

Aorto- refers to the aorta and *–plasty* means to form or reconstruct.

9.17

Angiostenosis is when blood vessels become too narrow.

Angiostenosis is made of three word forms: *angio-*, meaning blood vessels; *steno-*, meaning to make narrow; and *-osis*, meaning condition.

QUICK QUIZ *(Answers in Appendix A)*	
_____ 9.9 Lumen	*A.* The space within an artery
_____ 9.10 Fistula	*B.* An abnormal widening of a blood vessel
_____ 9.11 Embolism	*C.* Tube like passage from a normal vessel to another
_____ 9.12 Aneurysm	*D.* A vessel is blocked or stopped up

9.18

The next patient Dr. Sharp sees has a problem with his veins narrowing. What is the name of this condition?

_____ Phlebostenosis   _____ Myocardial ischemia   _____ Arteriovenous fistula

9.19

Dr. Sharp sees a patient who has chronic gastrointestinal ischemia syndrome. The opening to her celiac artery is filled with atheromas that are blocking the vessel. How would you describe this condition?

_____ Too much blood going to the stomach
_____ Abnormal opening of the artery
_____ Not enough blood going to the stomach

9.20

To correct the ischemia, Dr. Sharp removed a portion of the inner wall of the aortic intima and the lesions in the celiac artery. What is the name of this procedure?

_____ Angioplasty   _____ Endarterectomy   _____ Embolectomy

9.21

You've got this! Let's see how much word power you've developed. Here's a medical term we haven't shown you yet, but you'll be able to decipher its meaning. What is the meaning of renovascular?
(*reno- + -vascular*)

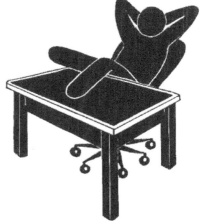

_____

9.18

Phlebostenosis is the narrowing of the space within the veins through which the blood flows.

Phlebo- is the Greek word for vein. *Sten-* means to make narrow; *-osis* means condition.

9.19

Chronic gastrointestinal ischemia syndrome is a deficiency of blood supply to the stomach. Ischemia is a deficiency of blood supply to an organ or part of the body.

Ischemia is made up of two Greek words: *ischein-*, meaning to hold back and *-haima*, meaning blood. It is to literally hold back blood from a body part.

9.20

An endarterectomy is the removal of the inner wall of the artery as well as lesions that have thickened the walls.

Endarterectomy is made of three word parts: *endo-*, meaning inner; *arter-*, meaning artery; and *-ectomy*, meaning surgical removal.

9.21

Renovascular refers to the kidneys and their blood vessels.

Reno- means kidney; *-vascular* refers to the blood vessels.

QUICK QUIZ (Answers in Appendix A)

_____ 9.13 Thrombectomy	**A.** Surgical removal of an embolus, material blocking a blood vessel
_____ 9.14 Embolectomy	**B.** Surgical removal of a blood clot
_____ 9.15 Transluminal atherectomy	**C.** Removing a blood clot and the inner wall of the artery
_____ 9.16 Thromboendarterectomy	**D.** Procedure to remove plaque from the arterial wall

Chapter Quiz 1 (Answers in Appendix A)

Choose the correct match.

_____ 9.1 Blood vessels with narrowed lumen	A. Angiostenosis
_____ 9.2 Inflammation of the aorta	B. Aneurysm
_____ 9.3 Repair/reconstruction of the aorta	C. Aortitis
_____ 9.4 Blood clot	D. Thrombosis
_____ 9.5 Formation/existence of a blood clot	E. Aortoplasty
_____ 9.6 A widened, weakened blood vessel wall	F. Thromboendarterectomy
_____ 9.7 Inflammation and blood clot within a vein	G. Embolism
_____ 9.8 Something blocking a blood vessel	H. *Thrombo-*
_____ 9.9 Removal of clot and inner wall of vessel	I. Thrombectomy
_____ 9.10 The surgical removal of a blood clot	J. Thrombophlebitis

You've got this! Use your new knowledge to decipher these words.

_____ 9.11 Thromboangiitis	A. Concerning the kidneys and stomach
_____ 9.12 Thromboarteritis	B. Any disease of the kidneys
_____ 9.13 Thromboendocarditis	C. Inflammation of blood vessel with a clot
_____ 9.14 Renography	D. Formation of a clot on inflamed surface of a heart valve
_____ 9.15 Renocutaneous	E. X-raying the kidney
_____ 9.16 Renogastric	F. Inflammation of an artery with a clot
_____ 9.17 Renointestinal	G. Concerning the kidneys and skin
_____ 9.18 Renopathy	H. Concerning the kidneys and intestine

Write-in the correct word from the list below.

9.19 A disease affecting the kidneys
        and their blood vessels _____

9.20 Removal of plaque on vessel wall _____

9.21 Within the thorax _____

9.22 Surgical removal of inner artery wall _____

9.23 The thickening of a vessel's inside wall _____

9.24 Deficiency of blood to a body part _____

9.25 The space inside a blood vessel _____

9.26 Veins with narrowed lumen _____

9.27 Any material that is blocking a blood vessel _____

9.28 The surgical removal of an embolus _____

Phlebostenosis	Ischemia	Intrathoracic
Atherosclerosis	Transluminal atherectomy	Embolus
Embolectomy	Endarterectomy	Renovascular disease
Lumen		

Chapter Quiz 2 (Answers in Appendix A)

Choose the correct match.

_____ 9.29 Lumen	A. The space inside a blood vessel
_____ 9.30 Intrathoracic	B. Veins with narrowed lumen
_____ 9.31 Renovascular disease	C. Any material that is blocking a blood vessel
_____ 9.32 Ischemia	D. Deficiency of blood to a body part
_____ 9.33 Phlebostenosis	E. Surgical removal of inner artery wall
_____ 9.34 Endarterectomy	F. The surgical removal of an embolus
_____ 9.35 Atherosclerosis	G. A disease affecting the kidneys & their vessels
_____ 9.36 Transluminal atherectomy	H. Removal of plaque on vessel wall
_____ 9.37 Embolus	I. The thickening of a vessel's inside wall
_____ 9.38 Embolectomy	J. Within the thorax

You've got this! Use your new knowledge to decipher these words.

_____ 9.39 Hepatalgia	A. Related to the liver and intestines
_____ 9.40 Hepatogastric	B. Swelling of a joint
_____ 9.41 Hepatoenteric	C. Surgically forming an opening into the bronchus
9.42 Hepatocele	D. Pain in the liver
_____ 9.43 Bronchocele	E. Surgically forming an opening into a joint
_____ 9.44 Bronchostomy	F. Swelling of the liver
_____ 9.45 Arthrocele	G. Swelling of the windpipe
_____ 9.46 Arthrostomy	H. Referring to the liver and stomach

Write-in the correct word from the list below.

9.47 Something blocking a blood vessel _____

9.48 The surgical removal of a blood clot _____

9.49 Removal of clot and inner wall of vessel _____

9.50 A widened, weakened blood vessel wall _____

9.51 Blood clot _____

9.52 The formation/existence of a blood clot _____

9.53 Inflammation and blood clot within a vein _____

9.54 Blood vessels with narrowed lumen _____

9.55 Repair/reconstruction of the aorta _____

9.56 Inflammation of the aorta _____

Aneurysm	Aortitis	Angiostenosis
Embolism	Thrombosis	Thromboendarterectomy
Aortoplasty	Thrombophlebitis	*Thrombo-*
Thrombectomy		

10

Review:

What we've learned up to now

In this lesson, we'll review the word parts learned in the previous lessons. This will help keep it in your memory! You will see some new words but you will know all the word parts. Are you ready? Let's go!

10.1

Dr. Sharp sees a patient whose heart muscle is inflamed. What is the name of this condition?

_____ Cystitis   _____ Pericarditis   _____ Myocarditis

10.2

Dr. Sharp's next patient has an inflamed bladder. What is the name of this condition?

_____ Cystitis   _____ Pericarditis   _____ Myocarditis

10.3

A new patient came in today with an inflamed vein in the calf. What is the name of this condition?

_____ Pericarditis   _____ Phlebitis   _____ Angiitis

10.1

Inflammation of the heart muscle is <u>myocarditis</u>.

Myocarditis is made of three word parts: *myo-* , meaning muscle; *card-*, meaning heart; and *- itis*, meaning inflammation.

10.2

Inflammation of the bladder is <u>cystitis</u>.

Cystitis is made of two word parts: *cyst-*, meaning bladder; and *-itis*, meaning inflammation.

10.3

Inflammation of the vein is <u>phlebitis</u>.

Phlebitis is made up of two word parts: *phleb-*, meaning vein; and *-itis*, meaning inflammation.

QUICK QUIZ *(Answers in Appendix A)*

_____ 10.1 *Lipo-*	*A.* Veins
_____ 10.2 *Rhino-*	*B.* Breasts
_____ 10.3 *Phlebo-*	*C.* Nose
_____ 10.4 *Mammo-*	*D.* Fat tissue

_____ 10.5 Pericarditis	*A.* Inflammation of the pericardium
_____ 10.6 Vesicostomy	*B.* Inflammation of the pelvis of the kidney
_____ 10.7 Pyelitis	*C.* Surgical opening into the bladder
_____ 10.8 Anastomosis	*D.* Connection of two parts of the body through a surgical opening that joins the two parts or the creation of an opening in a body part

10.4

The next patient has an inflammation of the sac surrounding the heart. What is the name of this condition?

_____ Pericarditis   _____ Pyelitis   _____ Angiitis

10.5

Dr. Sharp diagnosed his new patient as having inflammation of the pelvis of the kidneys. What is the name of this condition?

_____ Trigonitis   _____ Pyelitis   _____ Angiitis

10.6

The next patient has trigonitis. What part of his body is affected?

_____ The kidney   _____ The heart   _____ The bladder

10.7

Doctor Sharp performs a procedure during which he creates a surgical opening, or connection between two structures. What is the name of this procedure?

_____ Anastomosis   _____ Fulguration   _____ Litholapaxy

10.8

Dr. Sharp created a surgical opening in the bladder. What did Dr. Sharp do?

_____ A septostomy   _____ A vesicostomy   _____ A pyelostomy

10.9

Dr. Sharp surgically made a new opening in the bladder and connected the ureter to the bladder through it. What did he do?

_____ ureteroneocystostomy   _____ ureteropyelostomy
_____ ureteroureterostomy

10.4

Pericarditis is the inflammation of the pericardium, the sac surrounding the heart.

Peri- means surrounding; *card-* means heart; and *-itis* means inflammation.

10.5

Pyelitis is the inflammation of the pelvis of the kidney.

Pyel- refers to the pelvis of the kidney; *-itis* means inflammation.

10.6

The trigone is part of the bladder.

10.7

Anastomosis is the connection of two parts of the body through a surgical opening that joins the two parts or the creation of an opening in a body part.

Notice *stom-*, which means opening, is contained in ana-stom-osis.

10.8

A vesicostomy is the surgical opening into the bladder.

Vesico- is the Latin word for bladder and *–stomy* means opening.

10.9

Ureteroneocystostomy is a procedure that connects the ureter to the bladder through a new surgical opening.

Ureteroneocystostomy is made up of 4 word parts: *uretero-*, meaning ureter; *neo-*, meaning new; *cyst-*, meaning bladder; and *-stomy*, meaning surgical opening.

Quick Review	
Pore = tiny opening	*Diverticula* = little sacs
Metro = to measure	*Fistula* = abnormal opening

10.10

Because of congenital problems, Dr. Sharp enlarges an opening in the heart wall. What's the name of this procedure?

_____ Septostomy   _____ Pericardiostomy   _____ Pyelostomy

10.11

Dr. Sharp sees a patient who is having problems because the openings in one of her heart valves are too narrow. What is the name of this condition?

_____ Phlebostenosis   _____ Ureterostenosis   _____ Mitral stenosis

10.12

To correct the problem, Dr. Sharp makes an incision into the mitral valve. What did the doctor do?

_____ Cardiotomy   _____ Valvotomy   _____ Septotomy

10.13

That afternoon Dr. Sharp saw a patient whose veins were becoming too narrow. What is the name of this condition?

_____ Phlebostenosis   _____ Ureterostenosis   _____ Mitral stenosis

10.14

Dr. Sharp requests a record showing the pressure changes in the bladder at various stages of filling. What did Dr. Sharp request?

_____ Cardiotachometer   _____ Cardiopneumograph
_____ Cystometrography

10.10

Septostomy is a surgical opening in the septum, the wall inside the heart that separates the heart chambers.

Septostomy is made of two word parts: *septo-*, meaning wall; and *-stomy*, meaning opening.

10.11

Mitral stenosis is the narrowing of the opening in the mitral valve, one of the heart valves.

-stenosis is the condition of making narrow.

10.12

Valvotomy is a surgical incision into the valve.

Valv- refers to a heart valve and *–otomy* is a surgical incision, to cut into.

10.13

Phlebostenosis is the narrowing of a vein.

Phlebo- means vein; *sten-* means to make narrow; *-osis* is the condition.

10.14

Cystometrography is the record of the pressure in the bladder as it fills with liquid.

Cystometrography is made up of three word parts: *cysto-*, meaning bladder; *metro-*, meaning measure; and *-graphy*, meaning to write.

QUICK QUIZ (Answers in Appendix A)

_____ 10.9 *Dys-*	A. Bone
_____ 10.10 *Uro-*	B. Diseased, difficult or bad
_____ 10.11 *Endo-*	C. Inside
_____ 10.12 *Osteo-*	D. Urinary tract

10.15

Dr. Sharp has an older patient who has been fainting. He wants to record her heartbeat for a month. What does he use to record it?

_____ Cardiotachometer   _____ Cardiopneumograph
_____ Cystometrography

10.16

Dr. Sharp is concerned about his patient because his heart is beating too slowly. What's the name of this condition?

_____ Tachycardia   _____ Bradycardia   _____ Myocardia

10.17

Dr. Sharp sees a new patient who has an abnormal opening between the bladder and uterus. What's the name of the condition?

_____ Vesicocutaneous fistula   _____ Vesicouterine fistula
_____ Vesicovaginal fistula

10.18

The next patient has an abnormal opening between an artery and a vein. What's the name of this condition?

_____ Arteriovenous fistula   _____ Nephrocutaneous fistula
_____ Pyelocutaneous fistula

10.19

You've got this! Let's see how much word power you've developed. Here's a medical term we haven't shown you yet, but you'll be able to decipher its meaning. What does urethromeatoplasty mean?

_____

10.15

A <u>cardiotachometer</u> is an instrument used to measure the heart rate over a long period of time.

Cardiotachometer is made of three word parts: *cardio-*, meaning heart; *tacho-* meaning speed; and *-meter,* meaning measure.

10.16

<u>Bradycardia</u> is a slow heartbeat.

Bradycardia is made up of two word parts: *brady-* meaning slow; and *-cardia*, meaning heart.

10.17

A <u>vesicouterine fistula</u> is an abnormal opening between the bladder and the uterus.

Vesico- means bladder; *-uterine* refers to the uterus.

10.18

An <u>arteriovenous fistula</u> is an abnormal opening between an artery and a vein.

Arteriovenous is made up of two word parts: *arterio-* meaning artery and *-venous* meaning vein.

10.19

Urethromeatoplasty is the <u>reconstruction of the urethra and the meatus</u>, the passage into the urethra.

Urethromeatoplasty is made up of three word parts: *urethro-* meaning urethra; *meato-* meaning passage; and *-plasty* meaning reconstruction.

Chapter Quiz 1 (Answers in Appendix A)

Choose the correct match.

_____ 10.1 Inflammation of the kidney pelvis	A. Atherectomy
_____ 10.2 Inflammation of the bladder	B. Pericardiorrhaphy
_____ 10.3 Air or gas in the sac surrounding the heart	C. Pyelitis
_____ 10.4 Inflammation of the heart valves	D. Cystitis
_____ 10.5 Inflammation of the triangular area of the bladder	E. Nephroureterectomy
_____ 10.6 Suturing of the sac around the heart	F. Myocarditis
_____ 10.7 Removal of anything that is blocking a vessel	G. Valvulitis
_____ 10.8 Removal of thick lesions that are inside a vessel	H. Embolectomy
_____ 10.9 Removal of a kidney and ureter	I. Trigonitis
_____ 10.10 Inflamed heart muscle	J. Pneumopericardium

You've got this! Use your new knowledge to decipher these words.

_____ 10.11 Gastralgia	A. Pertaining to the stomach and the liver
_____ 10.12 Gastrocele	B. Pain in the stomach
_____ 10.13 Gastrocolostomy	C. Involuntary contraction of the stomach muscle
_____ 10.14 Gastrocolotomy	D. Narrowing of the stomach
_____ 10.15 Gastrostenosis	E. Pertaining to the stomach and the skin
_____ 10.16 Gastrospasm	F. Incision into the stomach and colon
_____ 10.17 Gastrocutaneous	G. Swelling of the wall of the stomach
_____ 10.18 Gastrohepatic	H. Surgical procedure to establish an opening between the stomach and colon

Write-in the correct word from the list below.

10.19 Surgical cut into the heart wall _____

10.20 Surgical fixation of the urethra _____

10.21 Surgical fixation of the aorta _____

10.22 Removal of stones from the kidney _____

10.23 Surgical connection of ureter to small intestine _____

10.24 Narrowing of a blood vessel _____

10.25 Inflammation of a vein _____

10.26 Inflammation of the pericardium _____

10.27 A surgical incision into the valve _____

10.28 The narrowing of the opening in the mitral valve _____

Nephrolithotomy	Septotomy	Angiostenosis
Urethropexy	Aortopexy	Ureteroenterostomy
Mitral stenosis	Valvotomy	Phlebitis
Pericarditis		

Chapter Quiz 2 (Answers in Appendix A)

Choose the correct match.

_____ 10.29 Mitral stenosis	A. Removal of stones from the kidney
_____ 10.30 Aortopexy	B. The narrowing of the opening in the mitral valve
_____ 10.31 Pericarditis	C. Surgical connection of ureter to small intestine
_____ 10.32 Septotomy	D. Inflammation of a vein
_____ 10.33 Nephrolithotomy	E. Inflammation of the pericardium
_____ 10.34 Valvotomy	F. Surgical cut into the heart wall
_____ 10.35 Angiostenosis	G. Surgical fixation of the urethra
_____ 10.36 Urethropexy	H. Surgical fixation of the aorta
_____ 10.37 Phlebitis	I. Narrowing of a blood vessel
_____ 10.38 Ureteroenterostomy	J. A surgical incision into the valve

You've got this! Use your new knowledge to decipher these words.

_____ 10.39 Thrombogenesis	A. Enlargement of the liver
_____ 10.40 Hepatomegaly	B. Instrument for the examination of the colon
_____ 10.41 Proctotomy	C. Examination of the stomach and duodenum
_____ 10.42 Proctalgia	D. Pertaining to the heart and liver
_____ 10.43 Cardiohepatic	E. Incision of the rectum
_____ 10.44 Gastroduodenoscopy	F. The formation of a blood clot
_____ 10.45 Colonoscope	G. Blood in the sac surrounding the heart
_____ 10.46 Hemopericardium	H. Pain in or near the rectum or anus

Write-in the correct word from the list below.

10.47 Inflammation of the heart valves _____

10.48 Removal of thick lesions inside a vessel _____

10.49 Inflamed heart muscle _____

10.50 Inflammation of the triangular area of the bladder _____

10.51 Suturing of the sac around the heart _____

10.52 Inflammation of the bladder _____

10.53 Removal of a kidney and ureter _____

10.54 Removal of anything blocking a vessel _____

10.55 Air or gas in the sac surrounding the heart _____

10.56 Inflammation of the kidney pelvis _____

Pneumopericardium	Myocarditis	Valvulitis
Pyelitis	Cystitis	Nephroureterectomy
Pericardiorrhaphy	Atherectomy	Embolectomy
Trigonitis		

Word Tour 2

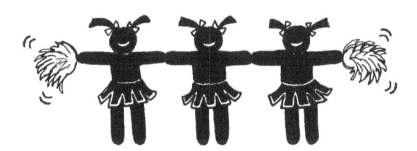

Congratulations! You've made it to the second Word Tour. Complete this and you will be half way to the finish! How are you feeling now? Are you getting confident in learning medical terminology? Take a moment to relax and pat yourself on the back.

Then, when you're ready, forge ahead to these review exercises. Working through these exercises will help you remember the things you've learned so far.

The questions are organized into two parts. You can work them one page at a time and check your answers with each page, or challenge yourself and check your answers after each part.

So, take a moment, then grab your pencil and get started!

NOTES...

Word Tour 2

Part 1 (Answers in Appendix A)

Match the definitions to the terms.

_____ 2.1 Surgery to reconstruct the aorta	A. Cardiotachometer
_____ 2.2 The surgical suturing of the sac surrounding the heart	B. Tachycardia
_____ 2.3 An instrument used to measure the speed of the heartbeat	C. Thrombophlebitis
_____ 2.4 Deficiency of blood due to a block in a blood vessel	D. Aneurysm
_____ 2.5 An inflamed vein with blood clot	E. Atherosclerosis
_____ 2.6 Removal of the inside artery wall	F. Pericardiorrhaphy
_____ 2.7 A weak, stretched spot on a vessel wall	G. Ischemia
_____ 2.8 A heartbeat that is too fast	H. Aortoplasty
_____ 2.9 An incision into the chest	I. Endarterectomy
_____ 2.10 Thickening of the walls of larger arteries	J. Thoracotomy
_____ 2.11 Abnormal opening between an artery and a vein	K. Myopericarditis
_____ 2.12 Inflammation of the heart muscle and surrounding sac	L. Arteriovenous fistula

Write-in the meaning of the term.

2.13 *Cyst-* = _____   2.15 *Vesico-* = _____

2.14 *Trans-* = _____   2.16 *Thoraco-* = _____

Match the definitions to the terms.

_____ 2.17 Reconstruction of a heart valve	A. Pneumopericardium
_____ 2.18 The narrowing of the openings in a heart valve	B. Valvuloplasty
_____ 2.19 Slower than normal heart beat	C. Pericardiectomy
_____ 2.20 Removal of a heart valve	D. Valvectomy
_____ 2.21 Removal of sac around the heart	E. Embolism
_____ 2.22 Reconstruction of the chamber wall in the heart	F. Mitral stenosis
_____ 2.23 Blockage of a blood vessel	G. Septoplasty
_____ 2.24 A procedure that uses the heart/lung machine	H. Cardiopulmonary bypass
_____ 2.25 Removal of blood clot and inner lining of a blood vessel	I. Transluminal atherectomy
_____ 2.26 Removal of lesions on the vessel wall by moving through its inner space	J. Bradycardia
_____ 2.27 Indicates an abnormal form, structure, or position	K. Thromboendarterectomy
_____ 2.28 Air or gas collected in the sac surrounding the heart	L. Anomaly

Write-in the meaning of the term.

2.29 *Renal-* = _____   2.31 *Brady-* = _____

2.30 *Tachy-* = _____   2.32 *Lumen-* = _____

Match the definitions to the terms.

_____ 2.33 Removal of anything blocking a vessel

A. Vesicocutaneous
   fistula

_____ 2.34 Removal of a blood clot

B. Cystolithiasis

_____ 2.35 Pertaining to the kidneys and their
       blood vessels

C. Hydronephrosis

_____ 2.36 Stones in the bladder

D. Meatotomy

_____ 2.37 Collected urine in kidney

E. Embolectomy

_____ 2.38 Swelling of the ureter near the bladder

F. Ureterocele

_____ 2.39 Crushing stones in the bladder and
       washing the fragments out through a
       catheter

G. Cystolithotomy

_____ 2.40 An incision into the passage into the
       urethra

H. Thrombectomy

_____ 2.41 Surgical connection of ureter and
       kidney pelvis

I. Renovascular

_____ 2.42 Inflammation of the bladder

J. Ureteropyelostomy

_____ 2.43 Fixation of urethra and bladder

K. Litholapaxy

_____ 2.44 An abnormal opening between the
       bladder and the skin

L. Vesicourethropexy

_____ 2.45 Incision into bladder to remove stones

M. Cystitis

Write-in the meaning of the term.

2.46 *-ologist* = _____   2.48 *-pexy* = _____

2.47 *-genic* = _____   2.49 *-cele* = _____

Match the definitions to the terms.

_____ 2.50 Inflammation of triangular section of the bladder	A. Nephrolithiasis
_____ 2.51 Surgical opening of the kidney pelvis	B. Trigonitis
_____ 2.52 Kidney stones	C. Pyelostomy
_____ 2.53 Destruction of tissue by high frequency electrical sparks	D. Anastomosis
_____ 2.54 Any surgery that approaches the organ through the urethra	E. Fulguration
_____ 2.55 Device for examining the urethra and the bladder	F. Endocarditis
_____ 2.56 The partial excision of an organ or a body part	G. Resection
_____ 2.57 Surgical joining of two structures or body parts	H. Cystourethroscope
_____ 2.58 Inflammation of heart's inner surface	I. Ureteroenterostomy
_____ 2.59 Connecting the ureter and small intestines through a surgically created opening	J. Transurethral surgery
_____ 2.60 X-ray of the bladder and urethra	K. Catheterization
_____ 2.61 Passing a tube through the body to evacuate or inject fluids	L. Nephroureterectomy
_____ 2.62 Surgical removal of ureter and kidney	M. Urethrocystography

Word Tour 2

Part 2 (Answers in Appendix A)

Match the terms to the definitions.

_____ 2.1 Aortoplasty	A. An instrument used to measure the speed of the heartbeat
_____ 2.2 Pericardiorrhaphy	B. Abnormal opening between an artery and a vein
_____ 2.3 Cardiotachometer	C. A heartbeat that is too fast
_____ 2.4 Ischemia	D. Thickening of the walls of larger arteries
_____ 2.5 Thrombophlebitis	E. A weak, stretched spot on a vessel wall
_____ 2.6 Endarterectomy	F. The surgical suturing of the sac surrounding the heart
_____ 2.7 Arteriovenous fistula	G. Inflammation of the heart muscle and surrounding sac
_____ 2.8 Aneurysm	H. Deficiency of blood due to block in blood vessel
_____ 2.9 Myopericarditis	I. An incision into the chest
_____ 2.10 Thoracotomy	J. Removal of the inside artery wall
_____ 2.11 Tachycardia	K. An inflamed vein with blood clot
_____ 2.12 Atherosclerosis	L. Surgery to reconstruct the aorta

Match the terms to the definitions.

_____ 2.13 Mitral stenosis

A. The narrowing of the openings in a heart valve

_____ 2.14 Valvuloplasty

B. Blockage of a blood vessel

_____ 2.15 Embolism

C. Abnormal form, structure, or position

_____ 2.16 Cardiopulmonary bypass

D. Removal of lesions on the vessel wall by moving through its inner space

_____ 2.17 Anomaly

E. A heart beat that is slower than normal

_____ 2.18 Transluminal atherectomy

F. Reconstruction of chamber wall in heart

_____ 2.19 Septoplasty

G. Surgical joining of two structures or body parts

_____ 2.20 Thromboendarterectomy

H. Removal of blood clot and inner lining of a blood vessel

_____ 2.21 Valvectomy

I. Procedure that uses heart/lung machine

_____ 2.22 Pericardiectomy

J. Reconstruction of a heart valve

_____ 2.23 Bradycardia

K. Removal of a heart valve

_____ 2.24 Anastomosis

L. Removal of sac around the heart

Write-in the meaning of the term.

2.25 *Pyel-* = _____   2.27 *Vasculo-* = _____

2.26 *Metro-* = _____   2.28 *Intra-* = _____

Match the terms to the definitions.

_____ 2.29 Catheterization	A. Pertaining to the kidneys and their blood vessels
_____ 2.30 Nephroureterectomy	B. An incision into the passage into the urethra
_____ 2.31 Transurethral surgery	C. Passing a tube through the body to evacuate or inject fluids
_____ 2.32 Resection	D. Surgical removal of ureter and kidney
_____ 2.33 Ureteroenterostomy	E. Removal of a blood clot
_____ 2.34 Endocarditis	F. Connecting the ureter and small intestines through a surgically created opening
_____ 2.35 Cystourethroscope	G. Partial excision of an organ or body part
_____ 2.36 Urethrocystography	H. Inflammation of the heart's inner surface
_____ 2.37 Renovascular	I. Stones in the bladder
_____ 2.38 Meatotomy	J. Collected urine in kidney
_____ 2.39 Hydronephrosis	K. X-ray of the bladder and urethra
_____ 2.40 Cystolithiasis	L. Any surgery that approaches the organ through the urethra
_____ 2.41 Thrombectomy	M. Device for examining the urethra and the bladder

Write-in the meaning of the term.

2.42 Stenosis = _____   2.44 Anastomosis = _____

2.43 Ischemia = _____   2.45 Resection = _____

Match the terms to the definitions.

_____ 2.46 Pneumopericardium	A. Crushing stones in the bladder and washing the fragments out through a catheter
_____ 2.47 Litholapaxy	B. Surgical opening of the kidney pelvis
_____ 2.48 Ureterocele	C. Air or gas collected in the sac surrounding the heart
_____ 2.49 Embolectomy	D. Removal of anything blocking a vessel
_____ 2.50 Fulguration	E. Inflammation of triangular section of the bladder
_____ 2.51 Nephrolithiasis	F. Surgical connection of ureter and kidney pelvis
_____ 2.52 Trigonitis	G. An abnormal opening between the bladder and the skin
_____ 2.53 Vesicourethropexy	H. Inflammation of the bladder
_____ 2.54 Pyelostomy	I. Destruction of tissue by high frequency electrical sparks
_____ 2.55 Cystitis	J. Kidney stones
_____ 2.56 Cystolithotomy	K. Fixation of urethra and bladder
_____ 2.57 Vesicocutaneous fistula	L. Swelling of the ureter near the bladder
_____ 2.58 Ureteropyelostomy	M. Incision into bladder to remove stones

11

The Respiratory System, Part 1: Breathe easy

Let's learn terms you'll use frequently if you work with information on the respiratory system. Some of these terms will be new; others will be old friends. First, let's look at the major organs included in the respiratory system. The major organs of the respiratory system include

The nose	The sinuses	The pharynx	The trachea
The larynx	The bronchi	The lungs	The pleura

11.1
Everyone knows where the nose is. Do you remember another name for the nose? What's another name for the common cold?

_____ Sinusitis   _____ Antritis   _____ Rhinitis

The paranasal sinuses are the ethmoid, sphenoid, frontal and maxillary. The sinuses are air pockets inside the bones. The names of the sinuses come from the names of the bones they are found in. One of their functions is actually to lighten the weight of the skull. They also provide mucus for the nasal cavity.

11.2
Which term refers to removal of cells in one of the paranasal sinuses?

_____ Sphenoidostomy   _____ Ethmoidectomy   _____ Maxillitis

11.3
Which term refers to a surgical opening into one of the sinuses?

_____ Ethmoiditis   _____ Sphenoidostomy   _____ Maxillitis

11.1

<u>Rhinitis</u> is an inflammation of the mucous lining of the nose. One type of rhinitis is also called the common cold.

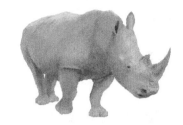

Rhin- is from a Greek word meaning nose.
-itis means inflammation.

11.2

<u>Ethmoidectomy</u> is the removal of cells from the ethmoid sinus.

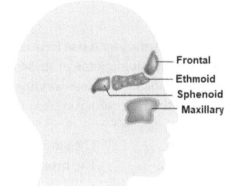

Ethmoid- refers to the ethmoid sinus and **–ectomy** means removal.

11.3

<u>Sphenoidostomy</u> is the surgical opening into the sphenoid sinus.

Sphenoid- refers to the sphenoid sinus and **–ostomy** means a surgical opening.

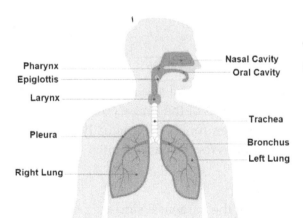

These are the other major organs in the respiratory system.

Here's some new terms we will learn.

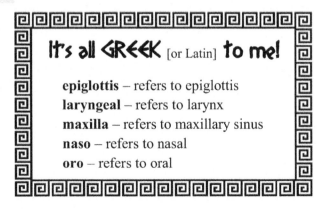

It's all GREEK [or Latin] to me!

epiglottis – refers to epiglottis
laryngeal – refers to larynx
maxilla – refers to maxillary sinus
naso – refers to nasal
oro – refers to oral

11.4

The pharynx has three parts: the nasal pharynx, the oral pharynx and the laryngeal pharynx. What's the oral pharynx called?

_____ Nasopharynx   _____ Oropharynx   _____ Laryngopharynx

11.5

At the opening of the larynx (also called the voicebox) is a leaf-shaped structure called the epiglottis. It covers the entrance to the larynx. When you swallow, it keeps food or drink from entering the larynx. When Dr. Sharp removes this structure, what is the operation called?

_____ Epiglottitis   _____ Epiglottidectomy   _____ Epiglottiplasty

11.6

Do you remember the names of the paranasal sinuses? Which of the following is NOT a paranasal sinus?

_____ Parotid sinus   _____ Ethmoid sinus   _____ Sphenoid sinus

There are three sinuses
shown in the illustration.

11.7
Label the maxillary sinus.

11.8
Label the frontal sinus.

11.9
Label the ethmoid sinus.

11.4

The oral pharynx is called the <u>Oropharynx</u>.

Take Note!

Oro- refers to oral. The pharynx's three parts are the nasal pharynx, or nasopharynx (*naso-* = nasal); the oral pharynx, or oropharynx (*oro-* = oral); and the laryngeal pharynx, or laryngopharynx (*laryngo-* = larynx). The pharynx begins behind the nose, extends behind the mouth, and behind the larynx.

11.5

The procedure of removing the epiglottis is called <u>epiglottidectomy</u>.

Epiglotti- refers to the epiglottis and *–ectomy* means surgical removal.

11.6

The <u>parotid sinus</u> is not part of the paranasal sinuses.

11.7

The <u>maxillary</u> sinus is located in the maxillary bone, the bone that forms the base of most of the upper face. Maxilla is Latin for jawbone.

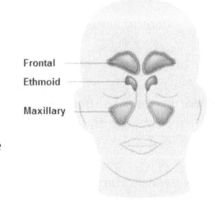

Frontal

Ethmoid

Maxillary

11.8

The <u>frontal</u> sinus is in the frontal bone, the bone that supports the forehead.

11.9

The <u>ethmoid</u> bone contains a number of sinuses.

Let's add these terms to your vocabulary.

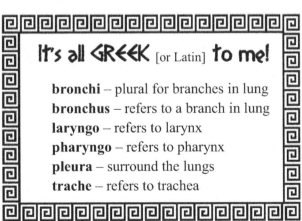

It's all GREEK [or Latin] to me!

bronchi – plural for branches in lung
bronchus – refers to a branch in lung
laryngo – refers to larynx
pharyngo – refers to pharynx
pleura – surround the lungs
trache – refers to trachea

11.10
Label the sphenoid sinus.

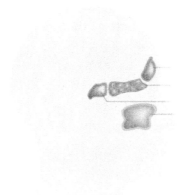

11.11
Gabby has a swelling in her pharynx. Dr. Sharp determines she has a hernia through the wall of the pharynx. What does Dr. Sharp call this condition?

_____ Pharyngography   _____ Pharyngocele   _____ Pharyngorrhea

11.12
Dr. Sharp orders an x-ray of Jose's larynx. What is another term for the record, or x-ray, of the larynx?

_____ Laryngography   _____ Laryngograph   _____ Laryngogram

11.13
Eddie needed an emergency tracheotomy performed. What did the doctor do when he performed the tracheotomy?

_____ removed the trachea
_____ made an incision into the trachea
_____ repaired the trachea

11.14
There are two branches of the trachea that carry air into the lungs. Look at the picture near the beginning of this chapter and write the name of these branches in the blank.

―――――――――――――――――――

11.10

The <u>sphenoid sinus</u> is in the cavity in the sphenoid bone, a large bone at the base of the skull, beside the occipital and ethmoid bones.

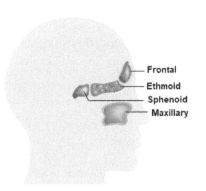

Now, you're familiar with the paranasal sinuses - the ones that communicate with the nose. Sometimes they're called the accessory sinuses.

11.11

This condition is called <u>pharyngocele</u>.

Pharyngo- refers to the pharynx and *–cele* means swelling or tumor. In this case, *-cele* is referring to the hernia.

The pharynx is a passage for both the respiratory and the digestive systems. When you speak, it also helps you form the sounds.

11.12

A <u>laryngogram</u> is the record, or x-ray, of the larynx.

Laryngo- refers to the larynx and *–gram* is the suffix for a written record, in this case an x-ray. A more common name for the larynx is voice box.

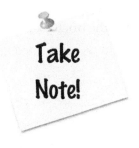

Take Note!

Remember: The suffix *–graphy* (Laryngography) indicates the procedure used to make the laryngogram and *–graph* (laryngograph) indicates the machine used to make the x-ray.

11.13

An incision into the trachea is called a <u>tracheotomy</u>.

Trache- refers to the trachea and *–tomy* means a surgical incision.

11.14

Each branch is called a <u>bronchus</u>.

Bronchus is singular; bronchi is plural.

11.15

Do you remember the Greek word for lungs? What is the name of the condition in which there is a hernia protruding from the lung tissue?

_____ Pyocyst
_____ Pleonasm
_____ Pneumatocele

11.16

The last major organ of the respiratory system is the pleura. Look at the picture near the beginning of this chapter and determine where the pleura are located.

_____ Inside the lungs
_____ Surrounding the lungs
_____ Throughout the respiratory system

11.17

The physician removes one of the sacs that enfolds the lungs. What's the name of this procedure?

_____ Pleurotomy   _____ Pleurography   _____ Pleurectomy

11.18

The physician removes the voicebox. What's the name of this procedure?

_____ Laryngectomy   _____ Epiglottidectomy   _____ Ethmoidectomy

11.19

The physician removes the structure that covers the entrance of the larynx when you swallow. What's the name of this procedure?

_____ Epiglottidectomy   _____ Pleurectomy   _____ Ethmoidectomy

11.20

Which of the following terms does NOT describe an inflammation of the sinus?

_____ Ethmoiditis
_____ Maxillitis
_____ Pleuritis

CLUE

Look back a few pages for the names of the sinuses!

11.15
<u>Pneumatocele</u> is the correct answer. *Pneumo-* is the Greek word for lung and *–cele* means swelling or tumor.

11.16
The pleura <u>surrounds the lungs</u>.

The pleura enfold both lungs. Always moist, they reduce the friction as you breathe in and out and the lungs expand and contract.

11.17
<u>Pleurectomy</u> is the removal of one of the sacs that enfold the lungs.

Pleura- is the name of the sac that enfolds the lungs. *-ectomy* is the suffix that indicates the surgical removal of an organ.

11.18
<u>Laryngectomy</u> is the removal of the larynx or voice box.

Laryng- is the root word for larynx, the voice box and *-ectomy* means the surgical removal of an organ.

11.19
<u>Epiglottidectomy</u> is the removal of the epiglottis.

The epiglottis is the name of the structure that covers the entrance of the larynx when you swallow. *-ectomy*, means the surgical removal of a structure or organ.

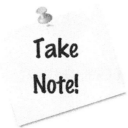

Take Note! Keep in mind the difference between *–ectomy* (excision), *–tomy* (incision) and *–stomy* (surgical opening).

11.20
<u>Pleuritis</u> is an inflammation of the pleura, the sac that enfolds the lungs.

Pleur- = pleura and *–itis* = inflammation. Ethmoiditis (*ethmoid-* + *-itis*) is an inflammation of the ethmoid sinus. Maxillitis (*maxilla-* + *-itis*) is an inflammation of the maxillary sinus.

Here's a few more terms to add to your knowledge.

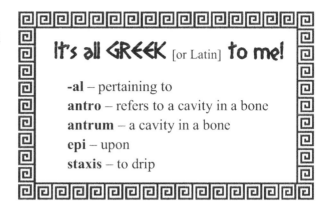

It's all GREEK [or Latin] **to me!**

-al – pertaining to
antro – refers to a cavity in a bone
antrum – a cavity in a bone
epi – upon
staxis – to drip

11.21

The patient has maxillitis. The doctor performs a Caldwell-Luc procedure, surgically opening a passage from the maxillary sinus into the nasal passage for drainage. What is the name of this procedure?

_____ Antrotomy   _____ Maxillectomy   _____ Thoracoscopy

11.22

To control a patient's hemorrhaging, the doctor ties, or ligates, the internal maxillary artery. To approach the artery, she goes through the maxillary cavity. What is another name for this cavity?

_____ Sinus   _____ Antrum   _____ Both sinus and antrum

11.23

The doctor approached the artery through the maxillary cavity. Which term below describes this approach?

_____ Transpalatine   _____ Transantral   _____ Transtracheal

11.24

A patient with sinusitis began hemorrhaging. What is the term for nosebleed?

_____ Rhinitis   _____ Pleurectomy   _____ Epistaxis

11.25

You've got this! What is pharyngitis?

_____

11.21

Antrotomy is the surgical incision into a cavity, in this case the maxillary sinus.

Antro- refers to antrum, a cavity in a bone. *-tomy* means a surgical incision.

11.22

Both sinus and antrum are names for the cavity in any bone.

11.23

Transantral means approaching through a cavity.

Trans- means through. *Antr-* describes the cavity, the antrum. *-al* indicates pertaining to or that this word is an adjective.

11.24

Epistaxis is another term for nosebleed. It is from a Greek word meaning to drip upon.

Epi- means upon; *-staxis* means to drip. When something falls in drops, this Greek term describes it.

11.25

Pharyngitis is the inflammation of the pharynx, or the throat.

Remember the pharynx is the tube that extends from the back of the nose to the larynx. *Pharyng-* = pharynx and *–itis* = inflammation.

QUICK QUIZ *(Answers in Appendix A)*

_____ 11.1 Phlebostenosis   **A.** The narrowing of a vein

_____ 11.2 Mitral stenosis   **B.** Inflammation of the pelvis of the kidney

_____ 11.3 Phlebitis   **C.** Inflammation of a vein

_____ 11.4 Pyelitis   **D.** The narrowing of the opening in mitral valve

---

Quick Review

Vasculo = refers to blood vessels	*Lumen* = space inside artery
Athero = fatty deposit	*Intra* = inside

Chapter Quiz 1 (Answers in Appendix A)

Choose the correct match.

_____ 11.1 A cavity, such as the sinus cavity	A. Pharyngocele
_____ 11.2 Leaf-shaped structure above voice box	B. Antrum
_____ 11.3 Swelling in the pharynx	C. Nasopharynx
_____ 11.4 Surgical incision into a sinus cavity	D. Transantral
_____ 11.5 Sacs that enfold the lungs	E. Epistaxis
_____ 11.6 The oral pharynx	F. Antrotomy
_____ 11.7 Nosebleed	G. Pleura
_____ 11.8 A hernia or swelling in the lung tissue	H. Epiglottis
_____ 11.9 Surgical approach through a cavity	I. Pneumatocele
_____ 11.10 The nasal pharynx	J. Oropharynx

You've got this! Use your new knowledge to decipher these words.

_____ 11.11 Nasogastric	A. Device used to see the nasal passage and pharynx
_____ 11.12 Nasopharyngeal	B. Concerning the nose and stomach
_____ 11.13 Nasopharyngography	C. Pertaining to the nose and pharynx
_____ 11.14 Nasopharyngoscope	D. Concerning the mouth and nose
_____ 11.15 Laryngopharyngography	E. Removal of the larynx and pharynx
_____ 11.16 Laryngopharyngectomy	F. Pertaining to the nose and trachea
_____ 11.17 Nasotracheal	G. Procedure for taking an x-ray of the nose and pharynx
_____ 11.18 Oronasal	H. Taking an x-ray of the larynx and pharynx

Write-in the correct word from the list below.

11.19 Removal of one of the sacs that enfold the lungs _____

11.20 Removal of the voice box _____

11.21 The procedure of taking x-rays of the larynx _____

11.22 Tube from larynx to bronchial tubes _____

11.23 Device for making x-rays of the larynx _____

11.24 Inflammation of one of the paranasal sinuses _____

11.25 An x-ray of the larynx _____

11.26 Inflammation of the lining of the nose _____

11.27 The two branches of the trachea
        that carry air into the lungs _____

11.28 Inflammation of the maxillary sinus _____

Laryngography	Ethmoiditis	Laryngograph
Bronchi	Maxillitis	Rhinitis
Pleurectomy	Trachea	Laryngogram
Laryngectomy		

Chapter Quiz 2 (Answers in Appendix A)

Choose the correct match.

_____ 11.29 Laryngography	A. Device for making x-rays of the larynx
_____ 11.30 Rhinitis	B. Removal of the voice box
_____ 11.31 Ethmoiditis	C. Tube from larynx to bronchial tubes
_____ 11.32 Laryngograph	D. The procedure of taking x-rays of the larynx
_____ 11.33 Laryngogram	E. The two branches of the trachea that carry air into the lungs
_____ 11.34 Maxillitis	F. Inflammation of one of the paranasal sinuses
_____ 11.35 Bronchi	G. Removal of one of the sacs that enfold the lungs
_____ 11.36 Trachea	H. Inflammation of the lining of the nose
_____ 11.37 Laryngectomy	I. An x-ray of the larynx
_____ 11.38 Pleurectomy	J. Inflammation of the maxillary sinus

You've got this! Use your new knowledge to decipher these words.

_____ 11.39 Laryngologist	A. Narrowing of the larynx
_____ 11.40 Laryngopathy	B. Incision into the larynx
_____ 11.41 Laryngostenosis	C. Establishing a permanent opening through the larynx
_____ 11.42 Laryngocentesis	D. Any disease of the larynx
_____ 11.43 Laryngitis	E. Hemorrhage from the larynx
_____ 11.44 Laryngorrhagia	F. A doctor who specializes in the larynx
_____ 11.45 Laryngostomy	G. Inflammation of the voice box
_____ 11.46 Laryngotomy	H. Incision or puncture of the larynx

Write-in the correct word from the list below.

11.47 Surgical approach through a cavity _____

11.48 Sacs that enfold the lungs _____

11.49 Leaf-shaped structure above voice box _____

11.50 Swelling in the pharynx _____

11.51 Nosebleed _____

11.52 Removal of voice box and throat _____

11.53 The nasal pharynx _____

11.54 Surgical incision into a sinus cavity _____

11.55 A hernia or swelling in the lung tissue _____

11.56 A cavity, such as the sinus cavity _____

Laryngopharyngectomy	Pneumatocele	Antrum
Nasopharynx	Pleura	Transantral
Epistaxis	Antrotomy	Epiglottis
Pharyngocele		

12

The Respiratory System, Part 2: The details will leave you breathless

We're going to spend a little more time going over terms of the respiratory system. Let's look at the larynx, the voice box, in a little more detail. You already know that its entrance is protected by the epiglottis.

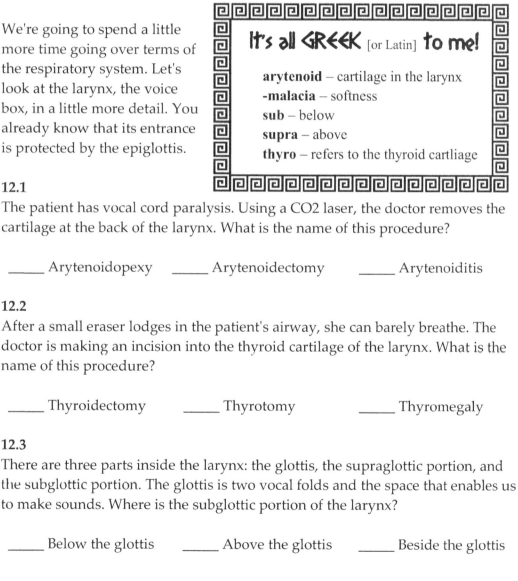

It's all GREEK [or Latin] **to me!**

arytenoid – cartilage in the larynx
-malacia – softness
sub – below
supra – above
thyro – refers to the thyroid cartilage

12.1

The patient has vocal cord paralysis. Using a CO2 laser, the doctor removes the cartilage at the back of the larynx. What is the name of this procedure?

_____ Arytenoidopexy   _____ Arytenoidectomy   _____ Arytenoiditis

12.2

After a small eraser lodges in the patient's airway, she can barely breathe. The doctor is making an incision into the thyroid cartilage of the larynx. What is the name of this procedure?

_____ Thyroidectomy   _____ Thyrotomy   _____ Thyromegaly

12.3

There are three parts inside the larynx: the glottis, the supraglottic portion, and the subglottic portion. The glottis is two vocal folds and the space that enables us to make sounds. Where is the subglottic portion of the larynx?

_____ Below the glottis   _____ Above the glottis   _____ Beside the glottis

12.1

Arytenoidectomy is the removal of the cartilage at the back of the larynx. The name of the cartilage the doctor removed is arytenoid.

12.2

A thyrotomy is an incision into the thyroid cartilage of the larynx.

Thyro- refers to the thyroid cartilage and *–tomy* means incision. Usually if the doctor is making an incision into the thyroid gland, the procedure is called a thyroidotomy, although it is possible to call it a thyrotomy. If you know the problem the patient is experiencing, you will know what part of the body the procedure refers to.

12.3

Subglottic means below the glottis.

Sub- means below and *–glottic* refers to the glottis. The subglottis portion of the larynx is the narrowest portion of the upper respiratory tract. Another example using *sub-* is subpleura. Subpleura means below the pleura (*sub- + -pleura*). Above the glottis is supraglottic (*supra- + -glottic*).

QUICK QUIZ (Answers in Appendix A)

_____ 12.1 *Rhino-*	**A.** Nasal, oral and laryngeal
_____ 12.2 Parts of pharynx	**B.** Ethmoid, sphenoid, frontal and maxillary
_____ 12.3 *Pneumo-*	**C.** From Greek word meaning nose
_____ 12.4 Paranasal sinuses	**D.** From Greek word meaning lung

Take a look at these medical terms. Then we will have some questions so you can practice using them.

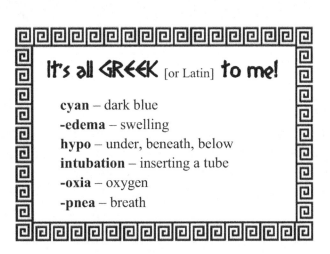

It's all GREEK [or Latin] to me!

cyan – dark blue
-edema – swelling
hypo – under, beneath, below
intubation – inserting a tube
-oxia – oxygen
-pnea – breath

12.4

The patient has bronchial stones. What is the term that Dr. Sharp will write in his notes for this diagnosis?

_____ Nephrolithiasis   _____ Broncholithiasis   _____ Bronchorrhagia

12.5

An infant is breathing noisily. The doctor diagnoses the problem as abnormally soft tissues of the voice box. Because the cartilage is too soft, the epiglottis is partially blocking the airway. What's the name of this condition?

_____ Laryngoparalysis   _____ Laryngomalacia   _____ Laryngocele

12.6

An infant is just recovering from a respiratory tract infection. He is having trouble breathing because of swelling in the subglottic region of the larynx. What is the name of this condition?

_____ Laryngoparalysis   _____ Laryngomalacia   _____ Laryngoedema

12.7

When the physician realizes his patient has laryngoedema, he immediately opens the airway by making an incision over the trachea and surgically creating an opening in the trachea. What is the name of this procedure?

_____ Laryngotomy   _____ Tracheoplasty   _____ Tracheostomy

12.8

A two-year old has had the flu. She comes to the doctor's office with subglottic edema, an inflamed trachea, and bronchi. She is having a difficult time breathing What is the name of her condition?

_____ Chronic   _____ Pneumopathy   _____ Laryngotracheobronchitis
        laryngitis

12.9

When a child has subglottic edema, the swelling may narrow a part of the larynx so that air cannot pass through. What term describes this narrowing of a passageway such as the larynx?

_____ Laryngospasm   _____ Laryngotomy   _____ Laryngostenosis

12.4

<u>Broncholithiasis</u> is the condition of having stones in the bronchus.

Broncho- refers to the bronchial tubes, *lith-* means stones and *–iasis* means the condition of. Put it all together and you have broncholithiasis.

12.5

<u>Laryngomalacia</u> is the softening of the larynx tissues.

Laryngomalacia is composed of two major root words: *laryngo-* refers to the larynx or voice box and *-malacia* refers to softness.

12.6

<u>Laryngoedema</u> is the swelling of the larynx.

Laryngo- refers to the larynx and *–edema* means swelling. Because the subglottic region is so narrow, a small amount of edema can block the airway.

12.7

A <u>tracheostomy</u> is a surgically created opening in the trachea that allows someone who has a blocked airway to breathe.

Tracheo- refers to the trachea and *–stomy* means surgical opening.

12.8

This term, <u>laryngo-tracheo-bronch-itis</u>, includes all three of the respiratory organs affected by the condition: the larynx, the trachea, and the bronchi. *-itis*, of course, indicates the inflammation and *laryngo-* refers to the larynx, *trachea-* refers to the trachea and *bronch-* refers to the bronchial tubes.

12.9

<u>Laryngostenosis</u> means the constriction or narrowing of the larynx.

Laryngo- refers to the larynx and *-stenosis* means the narrowing of a passageway.

Here's the last three terms for this chapter.

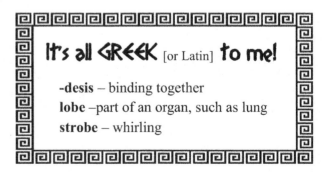

It's all GREEK [or Latin] to me!

-desis – binding together
lobe –part of an organ, such as lung
strobe – whirling

12.10

Dr. Sharp's next patient has symptoms that include hypoxia, cyanosis, and increasing tachypnea. What is hypoxia?

_____ Abnormally rapid   _____ Insufficient   _____ Bluish tint of skin
      rate of breathing   oxygen

12.11

What is cyanosis?

_____ Abnormally rapid   _____ Insufficient   _____ Bluish tint of skin
      rate of breathing   oxygen

12.12

What is tachypnea?

_____ Abnormally rapid   _____ Insufficient   _____ Bluish tint of skin
      rate of breathing   oxygen

12.13

To help his patient breathe, the doctor inserts a tube through the larynx airway. What is this procedure called?

_____ Endoscopy   _____ Intubation   _____ Laryngoscopy

12.14

The patient is having difficulty breathing. The doctor performs an endotracheal intubation. Where does the doctor insert the tube?

_____ In the throat   _____ Inside the larynx   _____ Inside the trachea

12.15

You've got this! Let's see how much word power you've developed. What is the meaning of hemothorax?

_____

12.10
Hypoxia means the <u>amount of oxygen in your system is below normal</u>.

hypo- meaning under or beneath or below; and *-oxia*, meaning oxygen.

Take Note!

Did you notice that both **sub-** *and* **hypo-** *mean under, beneath or below?*

12.11
Cyanosis indicates <u>bluish tint of skin.</u>

cyan-, means dark blue, and the suffix, *-osis*, means condition.

12.12
Tachypnea is <u>abnormally rapid rate of breathing</u>.

Tachy- means swift or fast; *-pnea* means breath.

12.13
<u>Intubation</u> is the process of inserting a tube into something, in this case, the larynx.

The word intubation, is made of in + tube + ation. *In-* means into. Tube means tube. *-tion* indicates the action or the process involved.

12.14
Endotracheal intubation is <u>inside the trachea</u>.

Endotracheal is made of a prefix, *endo-* meaning inside, and *trache-* indicating the trachea. *-al*, the suffix, makes the word an adjective.

12.15
Hemothorax is the condition of <u>blood accumulating in the pleural space in the chest</u>.

This word has two major parts: *hemo-* meaning blood and *-thorax* meaning chest.

12.16

The doctor wants to check the vibration of the patient's vocal cords. What instrument will he use?

_____ Laryngoscope   _____ Endoscope   _____ Laryngostroboscope

12.17

The doctor treated the problem by evacuating the blood before clotting occurred using closed tube drainage. She made an incision into the chest and inserted a tube. What is the name of this procedure?

_____ Thoracoplasty   _____ Thoracoscopy   _____ Tube thoracostomy

12.18

A patient has air accumulating in his pleural space. What is the name of this condition?

_____ Pneumothorax   _____ Hemothorax   _____ Hydrothorax

12.19

The doctor uses a needle to puncture the chest wall and remove the air. What is the name of this procedure?

_____ Thoracentesis   _____ Thoracoplasty   _____ Thoracoscopy

12.20

This patient has recurring pneumothorax. The doctor treats the recurrence by producing adhesions between the pleura to bind them together and stop any leaks. What is the name of this procedure?

_____ Thoracentesis   _____ Pleurodesis   _____ Tube thoracostomy

12.21

You've got this! Let's see how much word power you've developed. What is the meaning of lobectomy?

_____

12.16
Laryngostroboscope is an instrument used to view the movement or vibration of the voice box.

This word is made up of three parts: *laryngo-* indicating the voice box or the larynx; *strobo-* indicating whirling; and *-scope* which means to view.

12.17
Tube thoracostomy is inserting a tube into the chest.

Thoracostomy is made of two words: *thoraco-* indicating chest and *-stomy*, indicating an opening. In this case the opening is used to drain the blood from the pleural space.

12.18
Pneumothorax is air accumulating in the chest.

Pneumothorax is composed of two words: *pneumo-* meaning air; and *-thorax* meaning chest. Put these together and you get the accumulation of air in the chest, in this case, in the pleural space in the chest.

12.19
Thoracentesis is using a needle to puncture the chest wall.

Thoracentesis is made of two word parts: *thora-* indicates chest; *-centesis* means a puncture.

12.20
Pleurodesis binds the two layers of the pleura together.

This word is made of two words: *pleuro-* indicating the pleura; and *-desis* which indicates binding.

12.21
A lobectomy is the surgical removal of one lobe of the lung (*lobe-* + *-ectomy*).

The lungs are divided into three lobes: the superior, middle, and inferior lobes. Pneumonectomy is the term used when an entire lung is removed. When only a lobe is removed it is called a lobectomy. Sometimes the doctor will remove only one segment of a lung. This is called segmental resection.

Chapter Quiz 1 (Answers in Appendix A)

Choose the correct match.

_____ 12.1 Surgical excision of part of the lung	A. Thoracentesis
_____ 12.2 Incision into the thyroid cartilage of the larynx	B. Laryngotracheobronchitis
_____ 12.3 A surgical opening into the chest wall	C. Thyrotomy
_____ 12.4 Surgical binding of the pleural layers	D. Pleurodesis
_____ 12.5 Narrowing of the larynx	E. Thoracostomy
_____ 12.6 The softening of the tissue of the voice box	F. Tracheotomy
_____ 12.7 A faster than normal rate of breathing	G. Tachypnea
_____ 12.8 A surgical incision into the trachea	H. Lobectomy
_____ 12.9 A puncture, using a needle, into the chest	I. Laryngostenosis
_____ 12.10 Inflammation of the larynx, the trachea, and the bronchi	J. Laryngomalacia

You've got this! Use your new knowledge to decipher these words.

_____ 12.11 Subcutaneous	A. Beneath the pericardium
_____ 12.12 Submandibular	B. Decreased rate of breathing
_____ 12.13 Subpericardial	C. Surgical repair of the voice box
_____ 12.14 Subendocardial	D. Inflammation of the kidney due to stones
_____ 12.15 Hypopnea	E. Beneath the skin
_____ 12.16 Laryngoplasty	F. Incision of kidney for removal of stones
_____ 12.17 Lithonephritis	G. Beneath the endocardium
_____ 12.18 Lithonephrotomy	H. Below the mandible

Write-in the correct word from the list below.

12.19 Air pockets in the chest _____

12.20 Swelling of the tissue of the voice box _____

12.21 The act of inserting a tube _____

12.22 Above the glottis _____

12.23 Creating an opening into the trachea surgically _____

12.24 Insufficient oxygen _____

12.25 Surgical excision of cartilage of the larynx _____

12.26 Incision into the thyroid gland _____

12.27 Inside the trachea _____

12.28 Bluish tint of skin _____

Thyroidotomy	Tracheostomy	Intubation
Arytenoidectomy	Cyanosis	Supraglottic
Pneumothorax	Laryngoedema	Endotracheal
Hypoxia		

Chapter Quiz 2 (Answers in Appendix A)

Choose the correct match.

_____ 12.29 Intubation	A. Air pockets in the chest
_____ 12.30 Endotracheal	B. Bluish tint of skin
_____ 12.31 Tracheostomy	C. The act of inserting a tube
_____ 12.32 Arytenoidectomy	D. Surgical excision of cartilage of the larynx
_____ 12.33 Supraglottic	E. Swelling of the tissue of the voice box
_____ 12.34 Pneumothorax	F. Inside the trachea
_____ 12.35 Thyroidotomy	G. Creating an opening into the trachea surgically
_____ 12.36 Laryngoedema	H. Incision into the thyroid gland
_____ 12.37 Cyanosis	I. Insufficient oxygen
_____ 12.38 Hypoxia	J. Above the glottis

You've got this! Use your new knowledge to decipher these words.

_____ 12.39 Subrenal	A. Above the kidney
_____ 12.40 Suprarenal	B. Concerning the mouth and pharynx
_____ 12.41 Subhepatic	C. Above the liver
_____ 12.42 Suprahepatic	D. Concerning the mouth and face
_____ 12.43 Oropharyngeal	E. Pertaining to the larynx and pharynx
_____ 12.44 Orofacial	F. Below the kidney
_____ 12.45 Laryngopharyngeal	G. Inflammation of the larynx and pharynx
_____ 12.46 Laryngopharyngitis	H. Below the liver

Write-in the correct word from the list below.

12.47 Surgical excision of part of the lung _____

12.48 A puncture, using a needle, into the chest _____

12.49 Surgical repair of the voice box _____

12.50 A surgical opening into the chest wall _____

12.51 A surgical incision into the trachea _____

12.52 The softening of the tissue of the voice box _____

12.53 Inflammation of the larynx, trachea, and bronchi _____

12.54 A faster than normal rate of breathing _____

12.55 Narrowing of the larynx _____

12.56 Surgical binding of the pleural layers _____

Tracheotomy	Laryngostenosis	Laryngotracheobronchitis
Thoracentesis	Lobectomy	Thoracostomy
Tachypnea	Pleurodesis	Laryngoplasty
Laryngomalacia		

13

The Ear:

A real earful

Let's begin our journey into
the ear with these three terms.

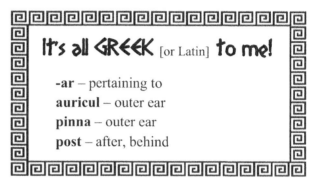

It's all GREEK [or Latin] to me!

-ar – pertaining to
auricul – outer ear
pinna – outer ear
post – after, behind

Are you familiar with the
parts of the ear? There are
three major parts of the ear:
the inner ear, the middle ear
and the outer ear.

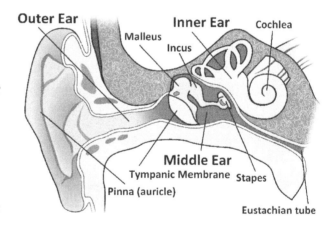

13.1
Which one of the parts of
the ear listed below is a part
of the outer ear?

_____ The stapes   _____ The mastoid process   _____ The pinna

13.2
The patient has developed a postauricular fistula. Where is this abnormal
opening?

_____ Inside the pinna   _____ Behind the pinna   _____ Inside the external
auditory canal

13.1

The <u>pinna</u> is the exterior part of the ear. Another term for it is auricle.

Pinna is from the Latin word meaning feather. The outer ear, like a feather, is a protruding appendage.

13.2

Postauricular means <u>behind the pinna</u>. Remember, another word for pinna is auricle.

Postauricular has three word parts: *post-* which means after or behind; *auricul-* indicating auricle; and *-ar* meaning pertaining to.

QUICK QUIZ *(Answers in Appendix A)*

_____ 13.1 Urethrocystography

_____ 13.2 Cystourethroscopy

_____ 13.3 Nephroureterectomy

_____ 13.4 Ureterolithotomy

A. The technique of x-raying the bladder and the urethra

B. Incision to remove stones from ureter

C. Using an endoscope to treat a problem in the bladder, or other body part through the bladder and urethra

D. Surgical removal of kidney and ureter

Here's a list of some more words we will cover in this chapter.

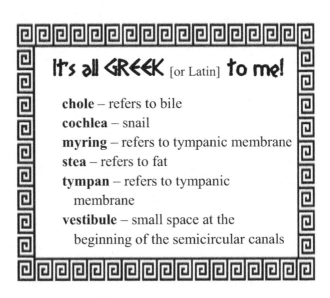

It's all GREEK [or Latin] **to me!**

chole – refers to bile

cochlea – snail

myring – refers to tympanic membrane

stea – refers to fat

tympan – refers to tympanic membrane

vestibule – small space at the beginning of the semicircular canals

13.3
What is the term for surgically suturing the meatus, the ear canal?

_____ Meatoplasty   _____ Meatorrhaphy   _____ Meatotomy

13.4
The patient has had a severe blow to his head. The doctor must reconstruct the external auditory canal. What is the name for this procedure?

_____ Otoplasty   _____ Tympanoplasty   _____ Meatoplasty

13.5
Meatoplasty is one term for reconstructing the external auditory canal. What is another term?

_____ Otoplasty   _____ Angioplasty   _____ Canalplasty

13.6
A child is born with lop ear, a deformity of the auricle. The outer ear protrudes too much. When the child is 6 years old, the doctor surgically reduces the cartilage protruding. What is the name of this procedure?

_____ Otoplasty   _____ Angioplasty   _____ Canalplasty

13.7
In the middle ear, there are three ossicles, tiny bones. Which of the following terms is not an ossicle?

_____ Malleus   _____ Incus   _____ Meatus

13.8
The patient is going deaf. The bones of the middle ear are hardening, becoming spongy. The stapes is becoming immobilized. What is the name of this condition?

_____ Otomalacia   _____ Otoneurology   _____ Otosclerosis

13.9
The doctor makes a small incision into the footplate of the stapes and inserts a Teflon wire prosthesis. What's the name of this procedure?

_____ Stapedotomy   _____ Stapedectomy   _____ Otoplasty

13.3

Meatorrhaphy is surgically suturing the meatus or external auditory canal.

Meatus means passage or opening (the eardrum to the external ear, or pinna). Meatorrhaphy has two parts: *meato-* the meatus and *-rrhapy* meaning suturing.

13.4

Meatoplasty is the surgical repair or reconstruction of the external auditory canal.

Meato- is from meatus, meaning opening or passageway and *–plasty* means surgical reconstruction or repair.

13.5

Canalplasty and meatoplasty are synonyms.

canal- a passageway or canal, and *-plasty* indicating repair or reconstruction.

13.6

Otoplasty refers to the reconstruction of the outer ear or auricle.

Otoplasty is made of two word parts: *oto-* indicating ear and *-plasty* indicating repair or reconstruction.

13.7

Meatus does not refer to an ossicle.

The malleus, the incus, and the stapes are the three ossicles found in the middle ear. These three bones transmit the vibrations from the eardrum, across the middle ear, to the oval window, the opening into the inner ear.

13.8

Otosclerosis is hardening of the bones of the ear.

Otosclerosis is made of three word parts: *oto-* indicates the ear; *scler-* means hardening; *-osis* indicates disease.

13.9

Stapedotomy is an incision into the stapes.

Stapedotomy is made of two word parts: *staped-* which indicates the part of the ear, the stapes; and *-tomy* which indicates the surgical incision.

13.10
Another patient with otosclerosis sees the doctor. This time to treat the disease, the doctor removes the stapes and replaces it with a prosthesis that he crimps over the incus. What's the name of this procedure?

_____ Stapedotomy   _____ Stapedectomy   _____ Otoplasty

13.11
Refer to the picture at the beginning of this chapter. What part of the ear separates the middle ear from the outer ear?

CLUE

It is also called the eardrum!

_____ The tympanic membrane   _____ The stapes   _____ The pinna

13.12
The patient has otitis media. The doctor makes an incision into the eardrum to aspirate the fluid in the middle ear. What is the name of this procedure?

_____ Tympanoplasty   _____ Tympanotomy   _____ Stapedotomy

13.13
What is another term that indicates a surgical incision into the eardrum?

_____ Tympanoplasty   _____ Myringotomy   _____ Stapedectomy

13.14
The auditory tube extends from the middle ear to the pharynx. The most important function of the auditory tube is to ventilate the middle ear space. What's another name for this tube?

_____ Eustachian   _____ Ossicle   _____ Meatus

13.15
The doctor must inflate the Eustachian tube. She makes a surgical incision into the eardrum and passes the catheter through the eardrum. What's the name of this approach?

_____ Transnasal   _____ Transtympanic   _____ Transmastoid

13.10

Stapedectomy is the removal of the stapes. Otosclerosis may be treated by stapedectomy or stapedotomy.

Stapedectomy is made of two word parts: *staped-* indicating the stapes, and *-ectomy* indicating the surgical removal of a body part.

13.11

The tympanic membrane (ear drum) sepearates the middle ear from the outer ear.

tympano- is from a Greek word meaning drum.

13.12

Tympanotomy is an incision into the eardrum.

Tympanotomy is composed of two word parts: *tympano-* referring to the eardrum, or tympanic membrane; and *-tomy*, meaning surgical incision.

13.13

Myringotomy is another term for surgical incision into the eardrum.

Myring- is the Latin word for tympanic membrane.

13.14

The auditory tube is called the Eustachian tube.

Eustachian comes from Eustachio, the last name of the anatomist who named the auditory tube. Another name for the Eustachian tube is otopharynx tube.

13.15

Transtympanic means through the eardrum.

trans- means through; *tympan-* means the eardrum; and *-ic* which means pertaining to.

Quick Review	
Thrombo- = blood clot	*Ren-* = refers to the kidney
Naso- = refers to the nose	*Oro-* = refers to the mouth

13.16

Because of pressure, a young boy's eardrum burst. The doctor repairs it. What's the name of this procedure?

_____ Meatoplasty   _____ Tympanostomy   _____ Myringoplasty

13.17

The middle ear is a cavity inside the temporal bone. What is the name of the cavity in the temporal bone that opens to the tympanic cavity?

_____ The pinna   _____ The mastoid antrum   _____ The ossicle

13.18

A woman has a problem hearing. She has a cyst-like sac, a tumor filled with epithelial cells and cholesterol, blocking the middle ear. The enzymes in the sac are eroding the ossicles. What is the name of this tumor?

_____ Otitis   _____ Cholesteatoma   _____ Otosclerosis

13.19

A patient has advanced middle ear and mastoid disease. The doctor removes the tympanic membrane, the ossicles and the cholesteatoma, and converts the mastoid air cells, the antrum, and the middle ear to an open cavity. What is the name of this procedure?

_____ Radical mastoidectomy   _____ Tympanostomy   _____ Myringectomy

13.20

The inner ear consists of a series of intricate communicating canals hollowed out of the temporal bone. What is the name of these maze-like canals?

_____ Stapes   _____ Ossicle   _____ Labyrinth

13.21

Part of the labyrinth is coiled, like a snail shell. It contains the organ of Corti, the receptor for hearing. What is the name of this part of the ear?

_____ Cochlea   _____ Meatus   _____ Auricle

13.16
Myringoplasty is repairing the eardrum.

Myringoplasty is made of two word parts: *myringo-* which means eardrum and *-plasty* which means repair or reconstruction.

13.17
The mastoid antrum, the cavity in the temporal bone, opens to the tympanic cavity. Remember from Chapter 11 that antrum means a cavity in a bone.

The mastoid is a portion of the temporal bone. It lies behind the external opening of the ear.

13.18
Cholesteatoma is a tumor filled with epithelial cells and cholesterol. Cholesterol is a normal part of bile. Remember *–oma* indicates a tumor.

chole- meaning bile, *stea-* meaning fat, and *-oma*, indicating a tumor.

13.19
Radical mastoidectomy is removal of the mastoid air cells and mastoid antrum.

Mastoidectomy is made of two words: *mastoid--* indicating the mastoid process, and *-ectomy* meaning the surgical removal of the elements named above: the mastoid air cells and the mastoid antrum. In this case, the removal of these elements creates an open cavity.

13.20
The labyrinth is a series of intricate communicating canals in the temporal bone.

The labyrinth contains the cochlea, the vestibule and the semicircular canals. One of its main functions is to maintain the physical equilibrium of the body. Another main function is delivering vibrations to the organ of hearing.

13.21
The cochlea is coiled and part of the labyrinth.

Cochlea comes from a Greek word meaning land snail.

13.22

Another part of the labyrinth is a small space at the beginning of the semicircular canals and behind the cochlea. What is the name of this part of the ear?

_____ Auricle   _____ Vestibule   _____ Pinna

13.23

What is another name for the acoustic nerve?

_____ Auricle   _____ Ethmoid   _____ Vestibulocochlear

13.24

The patient complains of constant buzzing sounds in her head. What is the name of this condition?

_____ Otitis   _____ Tinnitus   _____ Mastoiditis

13.25

Dr. Sharp must remove a patient's labyrinth. What is the name of this procedure?

_____ Labyrinthitis
_____ Labyrinthectomy
_____ Labyrinthotomy

13.26

You've got this! Here's a medical term we haven't shown you yet, but you'll be able to decipher its meaning. What is the meaning of tympanosclerosis?

_____

13.22

The <u>vestibule</u> contains an opening into the inner ear.

The three ossicles extend from the eardrum to the vestibule. The stapes connects to the vestibule. As in a house, the vestibule is the entranceway.

13.23

<u>Vestibulocochlear</u> is another term for the acoustic nerve.

Vestibulocochlear is made of three word parts: *vestibulo-* indicating the vestibule, *cochlea-* indicating the cochlea, and *-ar* which means pertaining to.

13.24

<u>Tinnitus</u> is constant buzzing sounds in the head.

Tinnitus comes from the Latin word for jingling. It may be caused by natural aging (presbycusis) or it may be symptom of a disease, like Meniere's disease.

13.25

<u>Labyrinthitis</u> is inflammation of the labyrinth.

Labyrinth- refers to the labyrinth and *–itis* means inflammation.

13.26

Tympanosclerosis is <u>hardening of the eardrum.</u>

Tympano- refers to the eardrum and *-sclerosis* means hardening.

QUICK QUIZ *(Answers in Appendix A)*	
_____ 13.9 Ureteroureterostomy	**A.** Joins the ureter and the sigmoid intestine
_____ 13.10 Ureterosigmoidostomy	**B.** Joins the ureter and the bladder
_____ 13.11 Ureteroneocystostomy	**C.** The joining of the ureter and the intestine
_____ 13.12 Ureteroenterostomy	**D.** The surgical joining of one part of the ureter to another part of the same ureter

Chapter Quiz 1 (Answers in Appendix A)

Choose the correct match.

_____ 13.1 Behind the outer ear   A. Meatus

_____ 13.2 Eustachian tube   B. Otopharynx tube

_____ 13.3 Hardening of the tissues of the ear   C. Mastoid antrum

_____ 13.4 A cavity in the temporal bone   D. Tympanotomy

_____ 13.5 Surgical repair of the ear   E. Pinna

_____ 13.6 Incision into one of the ossicles   F. Otoplasty

_____ 13.7 Passageway or cavity   G. Tympanosclerosis

_____ 13.8 Auricle   H. Postauricular

_____ 13.9 Hardening of the eardrum   I. Otosclerosis

_____ 13.10 Incision into the eardrum   J. Stapedotomy

You've got this! Use your new knowledge to decipher these words.

_____ 13.11 Tympanectomy   A. Occurring after hemorrhage

_____ 13.12 Tympanoplasty   B. Repair of the tympanic membrane

_____ 13.13 Posthepatitic   C. Instrument used for examination of the cardrum

_____ 13.14 Posthemorrhagic   D. Excision of the eardrum

_____ 13.15 Postethmoid   E. Occurring after hepatitis

_____ 13.16 Postpharyngeal   F. Behind the ethmoid sinuses

_____ 13.17 Myringectomy   G. Excision of the tympanic membrane

_____ 13.18 Myringoscope   H. Behind the pharynx

Write-in the correct word from the list below.

13.19 Intricate communicating passages in the inner ear _____

13.20 The eardrum _____

13.21 Reconstruction of the auditory canal _____

13.22 Approach through the eardrum _____

13.23 Tumor of cholesterol and epithelial cells _____

13.24 Ringing or buzzing sounds in the ears _____

13.25 Coiled part of the labyrinth _____

13.26 Removal of mastoid air cells and antrum _____

13.27 Inflammation of fluid in semicircular canals _____

13.28 Reconstruction of the eardrum _____

Myringoplasty	Transtympanic	Labyrinthitis
Cholesteatoma	Meatoplasty	Tympanic membrane
Mastoidectomy	Cochlea	Labyrinth
Tinnitus		

Chapter Quiz 2 (Answers in Appendix A)

Choose the correct match.

_____ 13.29 Tinnitus	A. Inflammation of fluid in semicircular canals
_____ 13.30 Labyrinthitis	B. The eardrum
_____ 13.31 Meatoplasty	C. Removal of mastoid air cells and antrum
_____ 13.32 Tympanic membrane	D. Intricate communicating passages in the inner ear
_____ 13.33 Myringoplasty	E. Coiled part of the labyrinth
_____ 13.34 Mastoidectomy	F. Approach through the eardrum
_____ 13.35 Cochlea	G. Tumor of cholesterol and epithelial cells
_____ 13.36 Transtympanic	H. Reconstruction of the auditory canal
_____ 13.37 Labyrinth	I. Reconstruction of the eardrum
_____ 13.38 Cholesteatoma	J. Ringing or buzzing sounds in the ears

You've got this! Use your new knowledge to decipher these words.

_____ 13.39 Postanal	A. Located behind the anus
_____ 13.40 Postcardial	B. Concerning the tympanic cavity and Eustachian tube
_____ 13.41 Tympanoeustachian	C. Deficient amount of menstrual flow
_____ 13.42 Vestibulotomy	D. Surgical incision into the vestibule of the inner ear
_____ 13.43 Hypomenorrhea	E. The science dealing with stones
_____ 13.44 Cyanuria	F. Below the urethra
_____ 13.45 Lithology	G. Behind the heart
_____ 13.46 Suburethral	H. Blue urine

Write-in the correct word from the list below.

13.47 Incision into one of the ossicles _____

13.48 Auricle _____

13.49 Surgical incision into the eardrum _____

13.50 Surgical repair of the ear _____

13.51 Behind the outer ear _____

13.52 A cavity in the temporal bone _____

13.53 Hardening of the tissues of the ear _____

13.54 Eustachian tube _____

13.55 Passageway or cavity _____

13.56 Hardening of the eardrum _____

Otopharynx tube	Tympanotomy	Stapedotomy
Mastoid antrum	Pinna	Otoplasty
Tympanosclerosis	Meatus	Otosclerosis
Postauricular		

14

The Mouth:

Mandibles, maxillaries and more

Let's start our exploration of the mouth with these three terms.

In the mouth, there are several structures that you

It's all GREEK [or Latin] **to me!**

cheil – lip
dent – refers to the teeth
labia – lip

need to be familiar with. The mouth, or oral cavity, includes the:

lips   uvula   palate   vestibule
tongue   salivary glands   dentoalveolar

14.1

What is a medical term for an inflammation of the lips?

_____ Cheilitis   _____ Cheilosis   _____ Cheilophagia

14.2

Charlie is having a surgical reconstruction of his lips. What is the name of this procedure?

_____ Palatoplasty   _____ Sialodochoplasty   _____ Cheiloplasty

14.3

What is another medical term that means lip?

_____ Glosso   _____ Lingua   _____ Labia

14.1

<u>Cheilitis</u> is inflammation of the lips.

Cheilitis is made of two word parts: *cheil-* is from a Greek word meaning lip; *-itis* means inflammation.

14.2

Surgical reconstruction of the lips is <u>cheiloplasty</u>.

Cheiloplasty is made of two words parts: *cheil-* is from a Greek word meaning lips; *-plasty* means the surgical forming or molding.

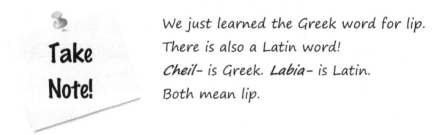

Take Note!

We just learned the Greek word for lip.
There is also a Latin word!
Cheil- is Greek. *Labia-* is Latin.
Both mean lip.

14.3

<u>Labia</u> means lips or a structure like one.

Labia is from the Latin word meaning lips. The singular word form is labium.

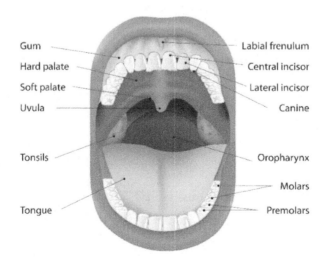

Gum — Labial frenulum
Hard palate — Central incisor
Soft palate — Lateral incisor
Uvula — Canine
Tonsils — Oropharynx
— Molars
Tongue — Premolars

Quick Review
Laryngo- = refers to the larynx   *Epi-* = upon or on top of
Trach- = refers to the trachea   *-staxis* = to drip

14.4

A patient has been in an accident. The doctor must remove the outside left border of the upper lip. What's the name of this procedure?

_____ Cheiloplasty   _____ Vermilionectomy   _____ Cheilitis

14.5

Dr. Sharp must perform reconstructive surgery on the roof of a patient's mouth. What is the name of this surgery?

_____ Palatoplasty   _____ Palatorrhaphy   _____ Palatoglossal

14.6

Which bone does NOT support the palate?

_____ Palatine bone   _____ Mandible bone   _____ Maxillary bone

14.7

Refer to the picture near the beginning of this chapter. What is the name of the small soft structure hanging from the soft palate above the root of the tongue?

_____ Salivary gland   _____ Uvula   _____ Tonsil

14.8

You've got this! Here's a medical term we haven't shown you yet, but you'll be able to decipher its meaning. What is the meaning of uvulopharyngoplasty?

_____

14.4

A vermilionectomy is the excision of the border of the lip.

Vermilionectomy is made of two word parts: *vermilion-* which comes from English and means bright red; and *-ectomy* which means surgical removal. The vermilion is the red boundary of the lips between the outer skin and the mucosa of the mouth. A cheilectomy is the excision of the lip, not just the border of the lip.

14.5

Palatoplasty is reconstructive surgery on the palate, the structure that separates the mouth from the nasal cavity. It's the roof of the mouth.

The front part of the roof is the hard palate, made from bone; the back of the roof is the soft palate, made of soft membrane. *Palato-* refers to the palate and *-plasty* means reconstructive surgery.

14.6

The mandible bone does NOT support the palate.

The palatine bone and the maxillary bone support the hard palate. Remember the maxillary bone? It's the upper jawbone. Palatine is the adjective form of palate. The palatine bone is the roof of the mouth and the floor of the nose.

14.7

The uvula is the small soft structure hanging above the root of the tongue.

Uvula is from the Latin word meaning "a little grape." The opening of the pharynx lies behind the uvula.

14.8

Uvulopharyngoplasty is the reconstruction of the uvula and the pharynx.

Uvulopharyngoplasty is made of three word parts: *uvulo-* which refers to the uvula, *pharyngo-* which refers to the pharynx, and *-plasty* which is the surgical forming or reconstruction of a body part.

Here's three more terms to learn about.

```
It's all GREEK [or Latin] to me!

alveo – refers to teeth sockets
gingiva – refers to the gums
sequester – to separate, isolate
```

14.9

What does *dent-* mean?

_____ the floor of the mouth   _____ the teeth   _____ the cheeks

14.10

What is the name of the part of the mandible and maxilla that contain the teeth sockets?

_____ Labia   _____ Palate   _____ Alveolar process

14.11

The patient has a neoplasm. The doctor must remove the part of the mandibular bone that provides the sockets for the teeth. What is the name of this procedure?

_____ Vermilionectomy   _____ Frenectomy   _____ Alveolectomy

14.12

What is the name of the part of the mouth that is outside the dentoalveolar structures, the part of the mouth that includes the mucosal and submucosal tissue of the lips and cheeks?

_____ Palate   _____ Vestibule   _____ Uvula

14.13

To help correct the deformity caused by cleft palate, the doctor reconstructs the opening in the mouth between the teeth and the lips. What's this procedure?

_____ Palatoplasty   _____ Cheiloplasty   _____ Vestibuloplasty

14.9

Dent- refers to the teeth.

14.10

The alveolar process contain the teeth sockets.

Alveolar is made of two word parts: _alveo-_ which is from the Latin word for small hollow or cavity; and _-ar_, a suffix which means pertaining to. The alveolar process is the part of the mandible (the lower jaw) and the maxilla (the upper jaw) that contains the bone sockets that the teeth fit into.

14.11

Alveolectomy is the surgical removal of the alveolar process.

Alveolectomy is made of two word parts: _alveol-_ refers to the alveolar process, the bone that provides the sockets for the teeth; _-ectomy_ indicates its surgical removal.

14.12

The vestibule is the part of the mouth outside the dentoalveolar structures.

A vestibule is a small cavity at the beginning of an opening. The vestibule of the mouth is the cavity between the inside of the lips and the teeth. This cavity forms when you close your mouth.

14.13

Reconstruction of the vestibule is called vestibuloplasty.

Vestibuloplasty is made of two words: _vestibul-_ refers to the cavity in front of the teeth, the vestibule; and _-plasty_ refers to the surgical forming of this part of the body.

Quick Review	
Sub- = below	_Supra-_ = above
-malacia = softness	_-edema_ = swelling

Here are a few more terms you
will become familiar with.

It's all GREEK [or Latin] to me!

gloss – tongue
hemi – half
ptosis – dropping

14.14

Which word refers to the teeth and the bone surrounding the teeth?

_____ Dentoalveolar   _____ Labia   _____ Vestibule

14.15

A patient comes to the doctor because of pain on his left side when he chews. The
doctor finds that the patient's gums are infected. What is this condition?

_____ Cheilitis   _____ Gingivitis   _____ Osteitis

14.16

A patient has severe dental pain. The doctor finds not only the gums but the bone
is inflamed. What is the name of this condition of the bone?

_____ Gingivitis   _____ Cheilitis   _____ Osteitis

14.17

The patient has severe gingivitis and some of the bone has died. As part of the
treatment, the doctor removes the part of the bone that has died. What's the name
of this procedure?

_____ Gingivectomy   _____ Cheiloplasty   _____ Sequestrectomy

14.18

Next, the doctor sees a patient with glossitis. What's wrong with the patient?

_____ His lips are   _____ His gums are   _____ His tongue is
    inflamed   inflamed   inflamed

14.14

<u>Dentoalveolar</u> refers to the teeth and the bones that surround the teeth.

Dento- comes from a Latin word that means tooth and *-alveolar* refers to the alveolar bone that surrounds the teeth.

14.15

<u>Gingivitis</u> is inflammation of the gums.

Gingivitis is made of two word parts: *gingiv-* indicating the gums, and *-itis* indicating an inflammation.

14.16

Inflammation of the bone is <u>osteitis</u>.

Osteitis is made of two word parts: *oste-* which refers to the Greek word meaning bone, and *-itis* which means inflammation.

14.17

<u>Sequestrectomy</u> is removing part of the bone that has died.

sequestr- which is from the Latin word meaning to separate and *-ectomy* which means to remove surgically.

14.18

Glossitis means an <u>inflamed tongue</u>.

Glossitis is made of two word parts: *gloss-* is from the Greek word meaning tongue, and *-itis* indicates an inflammation.

And, the last two terms for this chapter.

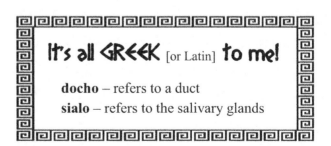

It's all GREEK [or Latin] to me!

docho – refers to a duct
sialo – refers to the salivary glands

14.19

An infant with cleft palate is having difficulty with the position of his tongue. It has dropped downward. When the infant is sucking, it can be sucked back and block the laryngeal airway. It is potentially life threatening. What is the name of this condition?

_____ Cheilitis   _____ Glossoptosis   _____ Gingivitis

14.20

A frenum, or frenulum, is a fold of mucous membrane that connects two parts. One of the parts is movable. The frenum keeps this part from moving too much. Frenum is from the Latin word for bridle. Which part of the oral cavity do you think has a frenum?

_____ the uvula   _____ the tongue   _____ the tonsils

14.21

The lip also has a frenum. What is its name?

_____ Sublingual frenum   _____ Labial frenum   _____ Buccal frenum

14.22

If the lingual frenulum is too tight, it's hard for someone to speak. This is commonly known as being tongue-tied. To correct this condition, the doctor makes an incision into the frenulum. What's the name of this procedure?

_____ Frenotomy   _____ Frenuloplasty   _____ Frenosecretory

14.23

Dr. Sharp performs a hemiglossectomy. What did he do?

_____ Surgical removal of the upper portion of the lip
_____ Surgical removal of half of the tongue
_____ Surgical removal of half of the cheeks

14.19

When the tongue has dropped out of position it is called <u>glossoptosis</u>.

Glossoptosis is made of two word parts: *gloss-* which indicates the tongue, and *-ptosis* which means "a dropping."

14.20

<u>The tongue</u> has a frenum.

The lingual frenulum extends from the floor of the mouth to the bottom of the tongue.

14.21

The frenum of the lip is called the <u>labial frenum</u>.

Labial means lip.

14.22

An incision into the frenulum is <u>frenotomy</u>.

Frenotomy is made of two word parts: *fren-* referring to the frenum, and *-tomy* meaning a surgical incision.

14.23

Hemiglossectomy is the <u>surgical removal of half of the tongue</u>.

Hemi- is a prefix that means half. *Gloss-* refers to the tongue. *–ectomy* is a suffix that means removal.

QUICK QUIZ *(Answers in Appendix A)*	
_____ 14.1 Myocarditis	*A.* Inflammation of the heart muscle
_____ 14.2 Cystitis	*B.* Inflammation of the pelvis of the kidney
_____ 14.3 Phlebitis	*C.* Inflammation of the bladder
_____ 14.4 Pyelitis	*D.* Inflammation of a vein

There are three kinds of salivary glands in the mouth

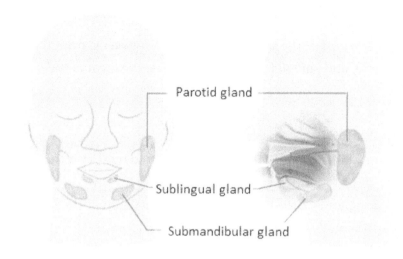

14.24

Sublingual tells you the location of the gland. What does sublingual mean?

_____ Below the jawbone   _____ Below the tongue   _____ Beside the tonsils

14.25

A patient has a small calculus in the sublingual salivary gland. The doctor removes the calculus. What is the name of this procedure?

_____ Sialodochoplasty   _____ Sialolithotomy   _____ Sialography

14.26

The doctor must repair the sublingual salivary gland. What is this procedure?

_____ Sialodochoplasty   _____ Sialolithotomy   _____ Sialostenosis

14.27

A doctor is repairing an abnormal opening between the lips and the nose. What is the name of this fistula?

_____ Nasoantral   _____ Nasopharynx   _____ Nasolabial

14.24

Sublingual means <u>below the tongue</u>.

Sublingual is made of three word parts: *sub-* means below, *lingual-* is from the Latin word meaning tongue, and *-al* tells you this is an adjective form of the word.

14.25

<u>Sialolithotomy</u> is the surgical incision into the salivary gland to remove a calculus.

Sialo- refers to the salivary glands, *lith-* refers to the calculus or small stone, and *-tomy* means a surgical incision. *Sial-* is from the Greek word for saliva.

14.26

Repairing the sublingual salivary gland is <u>sialodochoplasty</u>.

Sialodochoplasty is made of three major word parts: *sialo-* which refers to the salivary gland, *docho-* which refers to the duct of the salivary gland, and *-plasty* which means the surgical repair or reforming of the duct.

14.27

<u>Nasolabial</u> fistula is an abnormal opening between the nose and the lips.

Nasolabial is made of two major word parts: *naso-* which refers to nose, and *labia-* which refers to lips. A fistula is an abnormal opening between any two body parts.

Quick Review	
Hypo- = under, beneath or below	*Cyan-* = dark blue
-oxia = refers to oxygen	*-pnea* = breath

14.28

Label the parotid glands (try not to refer to the illustration on a previous page).

14.29

Label the submaxillary (submandibular) glands.

14.30

Label the
sublingual
gland.

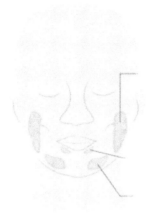
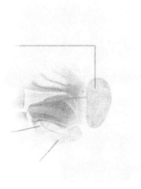

14.31

If a patient has a condition that involves the lips, tongue and the voice box, Dr.
Sharp might refer to this as:

_____ Sialoglossolaryngeal   _____ Palatoglossal   _____ Labioglossolaryngeal

14.32

If a patient has a condition that involves the palate and the tongue, Dr. Sharp
might refer to this as:

_____ Sialoglossolaryngeal   _____ Palatoglossal   _____ Labioglossolaryngeal

14.33

You've got this! Here's a medical term we
haven't shown you yet, but you'll be able to
decipher its meaning. What is the meaning of
sialolithiasis?

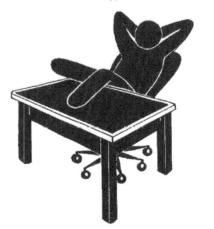

_____

14.28

The parotid glands are found in <u>the cheeks, in front of and below the ears</u>.

14.29

The submaxillary, or submandibular, glands are located in <u>the floor of the mouth</u>. They open where the frenulum attaches to the tongue.

14.30

The sublingual glands are <u>on the floor of the mouth, under the tongue</u>. There are several sublingual ducts which open near the tongue or into the submaxillary ducts.

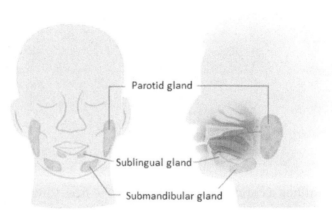

Parotid gland

Sublingual gland

Submandibular gland

14.31

The best response is <u>labioglossolaryngeal</u> (now that's a mouthful!).

Labio- refers to the lips, *glosso-* refers to the tongue and *-laryngeal* refers to the larynx or voice box.

14.32

<u>Palatoglossal</u> refers to the palate and the tongue.

Palato- refers to the palate and *-glossal* refers to the tongue.

14.33

Sialolithiasis is the condition of having <u>a small stone in the salivary gland</u>.

Sialo- refers to the salivary gland, *lith-* means stone and *–iasis* is a suffix that means the condition of.

Chapter Quiz 1 (Answers in Appendix A)

Choose the correct match.

_____ 14.1 Related to the teeth and the bone that provides their sockets	A. Palatoplasty
_____ 14.2 Inflammation of the lip	B. Palatoglossal
_____ 14.3 Relating to the palate and the tongue	C. Glossoptosis
_____ 14.4 Surgical removal of half of the tongue	D. Dentoalveolar
_____ 14.5 Excision of the outside border of the lips	E. Hemiglossectomy
_____ 14.6 Condition where the tongue drops downward	F. Cheilitis
_____ 14.7 Re-forming the roof of the mouth	G. Cheiloplasty
_____ 14.8 Surgical reconstruction of the lips	H. Vermilionectomy

You've got this! Use your new knowledge to decipher these words.

_____ 14.9 Alveoalgia	A. Removal of a section of the gums
_____ 14.10 Alveoloplasty	B. Pain in the socket of a tooth
_____ 14.11 Glossocele	C. Surgical repair of the tooth sockets
_____ 14.12 Glossospasm	D. Repair of fold connecting the tongue to floor of the mouth
_____ 14.13 Glossoplasty	E. An x-ray of a salivary gland
_____ 14.14 Glossorrhaphy	F. Narrowing of a salivary duct
_____ 14.15 Sialostenosis	G. X-raying the salivary gland
_____ 14.16 Sialogram	H. Suture of the tongue
_____ 14.17 Frenoplasty	I. Re-forming of the uvula, palate and throat
_____ 14.18 Sialography	J. A swelling of the tongue
_____ 14.19 Gingivectomy	K. Surgical repair of the tongue
_____ 14.20 Uvulopalatopharyngoplasty	L. Uncontrollable contracton of muscles of the tongue

Write-in the correct word from the list below.

14.21 Reconstruction of the opening in
the mouth between the teeth and the lips _____

14.22 Below the tongue _____

14.23 Reconstructing the uvula and pharynx_____

14.24 Condition of having a
stone in the salivary gland _____

14.25 Excision of the dead part of a bone _____

14.26 Relating to the lips, tongue and voice box _____

14.27 The inflammation of the gums _____

14.28 A fold of mucous membrane
that connects two parts _____

14.29 Repairing a salivary gland _____

14.30 An incision into the frenulum _____

Uvulopharyngoplasty	Vestibuloplasty	Frenotomy
Labioglossolaryngeal	Sublingual	Frenulum
Sialodochoplasty	Sialolithiasis	Gingivitis
Sequestrectomy		

Chapter Quiz 2 (Answers in Appendix A)

Choose the correct match.

_____ 14.31 Sublingual	A. Excision of the dead part of a bone
_____ 14.32 Frenulum	B. The inflammation of the gums
_____ 14.33 Sequestrectomy	C. Removal of a section of the gums
_____ 14.34 Gingivectomy	D. Re-forming of the uvula, palate and throat
_____ 14.35 Sialodochoplasty	E. Relating to the lips, tongue and voice box
_____ 14.36 Uvulopalatopharyngoplasty	F. Condition of having a stone in the salivary gland
_____ 14.37 Frenotomy	G. Below the tongue
_____ 14.38 Labioglossolaryngeal	H. Repairing a salivary gland
_____ 14.39 Gingivitis	I. An incision into the frenulum
_____ 14.40 Sialolithiasis	J. A fold of mucous membrane that connects two parts

You've got this! Use your new knowledge to decipher these words.

_____ 14.41 Sialolith	A. Pertaining to the tongue and palate
_____ 14.42 Glossolabial	B. Incision into the tongue
_____ 14.43 Glossopalatine	C. Pain in the tongue
_____ 14.44 Sialoadenitis	D. Study of the tongue
_____ 14.45 Glossalgia	E. Inflammation of a salivary gland
_____ 14.46 Glossopathy	F. A salivary calculus or stone
_____ 14.47 Glossotomy	G. Pertaining to the tongue and lips
_____ 14.48 Glossology	H. Disease of the tongue

Write-in the correct word from the list below.

14.49 Inflammation of the lip _____

14.50 Condition where the tongue drops downward _____

14.51 Excision of the outside border of the lips _____

14.55 Surgical reconstruction of the lips _____

14.53 Re-forming the roof of the mouth _____

14.54 Related to the teeth and the
        bone that provides their sockets _____

14.55 X-raying the salivary gland _____

14.56 Surgical removal of half of the tongue _____

14.57 Repair of fold connecting the
        tongue to floor of the mouth _____

14.58 Relating to the palate and the tongue _____

Glossoptosis	Hemiglossectomy	Palatoglossal
Dentoalveolar	Vermilionectomy	Sialography
Cheilitis	Palatoplasty	Frenoplasty
Cheiloplasty		

15

The Eye:

Oh, eye see

Are you familiar with the parts of the eye? Let's see. We'll start with these three terms.

It's all GREEK [or Latin] to me!

capsul – refers to the capsule of the lens

conjunctiv – refers to the conjunctiva

irido – refers to the iris

kerato – refers to the cornea

scler – refers to the sclera

15.1

The sclera is a protective covering of the outside of the eye. What is the name of the procedure that involves removing the sclera?

_____ Scleritis _____ Sclerectomy _____ Sclerostomy

15.2

Dr. Seewell's patient has a condition where the sclera is becoming thinner and softening. What's this condition called?

_____ Scleromalacia _____ Scleritis _____ Scleroplasty

15.3

The orbit is the bony cavity of the skull that contains the eye. You hear Dr. Seewell use the term orbitonasal. What does orbitonasal refer to?

_____ The orbit and the sinuses
_____ The orbit and the nose
_____ The orbit and the roof of the mouth
_____ The orbit and the tear glands

15.1

Sclerectomy is the removal of the sclera.

Scler- refers to the sclera and *–ectomy* means to remove. The sclera is commonly known as the "whites of the eye".

15.2

The best response is scleromalacia.

Sclero- refers to the sclera. *-malacia* means softening.

15.3

Orbitonasal refers to the orbit and the nose.

The parts of the eye:

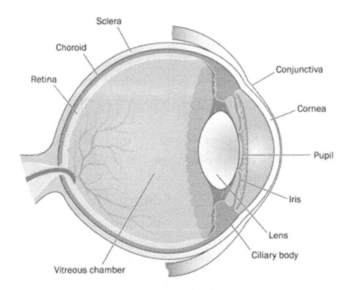

Here's some more terms that we will cover in this chapter.

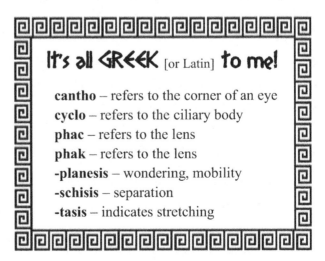

It's all GREEK [or Latin] to me!

cantho – refers to the corner of an eye
cyclo – refers to the ciliary body
phac – refers to the lens
phak – refers to the lens
-planesis – wondering, mobility
-schisis – separation
-tasis – indicates stretching

15.4

The iris regulates the entrance of light. Dr. Seewell must make an incision into a patient's iris. What does Dr. Seewell call this procedure?

_____ Iridoplasty   _____ Iridocyclectomy   _____ Iridotomy

15.5

Ricky has a condition where there is blood in his cornea. What is the name of this condition?

_____ Keratohemia   _____ Keratoiditis   _____ Keratomalacia

15.6

Lucy has a tumor in the conjunctiva of her eye. What does Dr. Seewell call this condition?

_____ Conjunctivitis   _____ Conjunctivoplasty   _____ Conjunctivoma

15.7

Fred has a condition involving the choroid. Which term below is a term that means any disease of the choroid?

_____ Choroiditis   _____ Choroidopathy   _____ Choroidocyclitis

15.8

Ethel has a condition where both the choroid and the retina are inflamed. What is the name of this condition?

_____ Choroiditis   _____ Choroidoretinitis   _____ Choroidocyclitis

15.9

Dr. Seewell must repair the patient's cornea. What is the name of this procedure?

_____ Keratotomy   _____ Keratoplasty   _____ Scleroplasty

15.10

What is the name of the condition when both the choroid and the ciliary body are inflamed?

_____ Choroidocyclitis   _____ Choroiditis   _____ Choroidoretinitis

15.4
Iridotomy is an incision into the iris.

Irido- refers to the iris. *–tomy* indicates the surgical incision.

15.5
Keratohemia means blood in the cornea.

Kerato- refers to the cornea. *–hemia* means blood. Put them together and you have keratohemia – blood in the cornea.

15.6
Conjunctivoma means tumor of the conjunctiva.

Conjunctiv- refers to the conjunctiva and *–oma* means tumor.

15.7
Choroidopathy means any disease of the choroid.

Choroid- refers to the choroid of the eye. *–pathy* means a disease. The choroid forms a dark brown vascular coat around the eye. Choroid is from a Greek word meaning skin like.

15.8
Choroidoretinitis is when both the choroid and the retina are inflamed.

Choroid- refers to the choroid. *Retin-* refers to the retina and *–itis* means inflammation.

15.9
The procedure of repairing the cornea is keratoplasty.

Kerato- refers to the cornea and *-plasty* means to repair.

15.10
Choroidocyclitis is when both the choroid and the ciliary body are inflamed.

Choroido- refers to the choroid, *cycl-* refers to the ciliary body and *–itis* means inflammation.

15.11

What's the term for surgical incision of the sclera and the iris?

_____ Scleritis   _____ Scleriritomy   _____ Keratoscleritis

15.12

Which part of the eye secretes tears?

_____ Orbit   _____ Lacrimal gland   _____ Choroid

15.13

A patient is considering plastic surgery because his eyelids are drooping. What is the name of this condition?

_____ Blepharorrhea   _____ Blepharoptosis   _____ Blepharostenosis

15.14

A patient has a problem with his eyebrow or forehead dropping. What's the name of this condition?

_____ Brow ptosis   _____ Sclerochoroiditis   _____ Keratopathy

15.15

Dr. Seewell must make a surgical incision into the eyelid. What's the name of this procedure?

_____ Keratotomy   _____ Blepharotomy   _____ Iridotomy

15.16

Dr. Seewell must make a surgical incision into the corner of the left eye. What's the name of this procedure?

_____ Keratotomy   _____ Blepharotomy   _____ Canthotomy

15.17

Dr. Seewell must make an incision into the patient's cornea. What is this procedure?

_____ Keratotomy   _____ Iridotomy   _____ Blepharotomy

15.11

Scleriritomy is a surgical incision of the sclera and the iris.

Scler- refers to the sclera, *iri-* refers to the iris, and *–tomy* indicates a surgical incision.

15.12

The best response is lacrimal gland. This gland is located in the orbit of the eye. One is above the eyeball and another beside the eyeball.

15.13

Blepharoptosis is drooping of the eyelids.

Blepharoptosis is made of two major word parts: *blepharo-* which means eyelid and *-ptosis* which means to drop.

15.14

Brow ptosis is when the brow drops or falls downward.

-ptosis means to droop, to move downward in position.

15.15

Blepharotomy is a surgical incision into the eyelid.

Blepharotomy is made of two word parts: *blepharo-* which refers to the eyelid and *-tomy* which indicates a surgical incision.

15.16

Canthotomy is a surgical incision into the canthus, the corner of the eye.

Canthotomy is made of two words: *cantho-* refers to the corners of the eye; *-tomy* indicates a surgical incision.

15.17

Keratotomy is a surgical incision into the cornea.

Keratotomy is made of two word parts: *kerat-* which refers to the cornea, and *-tomy* which indicates a surgical incision.

Quick Review	
Post- = after or behind	*Gingivi-* = gums
-desis = binding	*-iasis* = the condition of

15.18

The doctor must make a surgical incision into the iris. What is the name of this procedure?

_____ Keratotomy   _____ Iridotomy   _____ Blepharotomy

15.19

A young, malnourished child visits Dr. Seewell. Dr. Seewell finds that the tissue that makes up the cornea is softening. What is the name of this condition?

_____ Iridotasis   _____ Keratomalacia   _____ Blepharedema

15.20

A patient with glaucoma is seeing Dr. Seewell. He is stretching the iris as treatment. What is the name of this procedure?

_____ Iridocyclectomy   _____ Iridotasis   _____ Keratomalacia

15.21

Dr. Seewell sees a patient whose eyelids are swollen. The upper eyelid is baggy, hanging over the eye. What's the name of this condition?

_____ Iridotasis   _____ Keratomalacia   _____ Blepharedema

15.22

Dr. Seewell is operating to correct hyperopia, farsightedness. He removes the corneal epithelium and sutures on a new corneal tissue lenticule. What's the name of this procedure?

_____ Epikeratophakia   _____ Iridotasis   _____ Keratoplasty

15.23

Dr. Seewell sees a patient with hardening of the lens. What is the name of this condition?

_____ Scleritis   _____ Phacosclerosis   _____ Choroiditis

15.18
Iridotomy is a surgical incision into the iris.

Iridotomy is made of two word parts: *irid-* is from the Greek word meaning colored circle. It refers to the iris. *-tomy* indicates a surgical incision.

15.19
Keratomalacia means softening of the cornea.

Keratomalacia is made of two word parts: *kerato-* refers to the cornea and *-malacia* means softness.

15.20
Iridotasis is stretching the iris.

Iridotasis is made of two word parts: *irido-* refers to the iris and *-tasis* indicates stretching. When you think –tasis, think – t a s i s.

15.21
Swelling of the eyelids is blepharedema.

Blepharedema is a word made of two parts: *blephar-* refers to the eyelids and *-edema* means swelling.

15.22
Epikeratophakia is removing the epithelium and suturing a new corneal tissue lenticule.

The word epikeratophakia has three major word parts: *epi-* means on or upon and refers to the epithelium, *kerato-* refers to the cornea, and *phakia-* refers to the lens. Lenticule means lens shaped.

15.23
Hardening of the lens is phacosclerosis.

Phacosclerosis is made of two major word parts: *phac-* refers to the lens and *–sclerosis* means hardening.

15.24

Dr. Seewell sees a patient whose ciliary body and cornea are infected. What's the name of this condition?

_____ Phacomatosis   _____ Cyclokeratitis   _____ Sclerochoroiditis

15.25

Dr. Seewell must remove part of the ciliary body. What's the name of this procedure?

_____ Cyclectomy   _____ Phacosclerosis   _____ Sclerectomy

15.26

Dr. Seewell must remove the patient's iris and capsule of the lens. What's the name of this procedure?

_____ Cyclectomy
_____ Iridocapsulectomy
_____ Sclerectomy

CLUE

By now, "-tomy" is a no-brainer for you. Concentrate on the eye parts in the Greek/Latin box on page 221!

15.27

Dr. Seewell treats a patient who has an abnormal mobility of the lens. What's the name of this condition?

_____ Choroidopathy   _____ Phacoplanesis   _____ Phacomalacia

QUICK QUIZ *(Answers in Appendix A)*

_____ 15.1 Labial frenum   *A.* Inflammation of the gums

_____ 15.2 Lingual frenulum   *B.* Inflammation of the tongue

_____ 15.3 Glossitis   *C.* The frenum of the lip

_____ 15.4 Gingivitis   *D.* Extends from the floor of the mouth to the bottom of the tongue

15.24
Cyclokeratitis is inflammation of the ciliary body and cornea.

Cyclokeratitis is made of three major word parts: *cyclo-* refers to the ciliary body, *kerat-* refers to the cornea, and *-itis* means infection or inflammation.

15.25
Cyclectomy means surgical removal of the ciliary body.

Cyclectomy is made of two major word parts: *cycl-* refers to the ciliary body and *-ectomy* refers to its surgical excision.

15.26
Iridocapsulectomy is the removal of the iris and the capsule of the lens.

Iridocapsulectomy is made of three major word parts: *irido-* refers to the iris, *capsul-* means "little box" and refers to the capsule of the lens, and *-ectomy* refers to their surgical excision.

15.27
Phacoplanesis is an abnormal mobility of the lens.

Phacoplanesis has two major word parts: *phaco-* refers to the lens, and *-planesis* comes from the Greek for wandering and indicates mobility.

QUICK QUIZ (Answers in Appendix A)

_____ 15.5 Blepharoptosis	**A.** A surgical incision into the eyelid
_____ 15.6 Cyclectomy	**B.** Excision of part of the ciliary body
_____ 15.7 Blepharotomy	**C.** Drooping eyelids
_____ 15.8 Canthotomy	**D.** Surgical incision into the corner of the eye

_____ 15.9 Keratotomy	**A.** A surgical incision into the iris
_____ 15.10 Iridotomy	**B.** Softening of the cornea
_____ 15.11 Keratomalacia	**C.** Hardening of the lens
_____ 15.12 Phacosclerosis	**D.** An incision into the patient's cornea

15.28

A patient has a condition where the iris has separated into two layers. What is the name of this condition?

_____ Iridoptosis   _____ Iridoschisis   _____ Iridotasis

15.29

Dr. Seewell's next patient has an inflammation of the iris, the ciliary body and the choroid. What is this condition called?

_____ Scleromalacia   _____ Iridoptosis   _____ Iridocyclochoroiditis

15.30

Dr. Seewell has a patient whos iris has dropped out of its position. When Dr. Seewell writes in the patient's chart, what does he put down for a diagnosis?

_____ Scleromalacia   _____ Iridoptosis   _____ Iridocyclochoroiditis

15.31

Dr. Seewell performs an operation involving a cut into the lacrimal duct. What is the name of this procedure?

_____ Lacrimotomy   _____ Blepharotomy   _____ Keratotomy

15.32

You've got this! Let's see how much word power you've developed. Here's a medical term we haven't shown you yet, but you'll be able to decipher its meaning. What is the meaning of orbitotomy?

_____

15.28
Separation of the iris into two layers is called <u>Iridoschisis</u>.

Irido- refers to the iris and *–schisis* means separation.

15.29
Inflammation of the iris, ciliary body and choroid is <u>iridocyclochoroiditis</u>.

Irido- refers to the iris, *cyclo-* refers to the ciliary body, *choroid-* refers to the choroid and *–itis* is inflammation. Therefore, iridocyclochoroiditis (a big word indeed!) is inflammation of the iris, the ciliary body and the choroid.

15.30
<u>Iridoptosis</u> is the condition of the iris dropping out of position.

Irido- refers to the iris and *–ptosis* is the condition when something drops out of its position.

15.31
<u>Lacrimotomy</u> is the incision of the lacrimal duct.

Lacri- refers to the lacrimal duct and *–otomy* means surgical incision.

15.32
Orbitotomy is the <u>incision into the bone surrounding the eye.</u>

The orbit is the bony cavity of the skull that contains the eyeball. *–otomy* is the suffix that indicates an incision.

QUICK QUIZ *(Answers in Appendix A)*	
_____ 15.13 Blepharotomy	*A.* Stretching the iris
_____ 15.14 Blepharedema	*B.* A surgical incision into the eyelid
_____ 15.15 Iridotasis	*C.* Abnormal mobility of the lens
_____ 15.16 Phacoplanesis	*D.* Swelling of the eyelids

Chapter Quiz 1 (Answers in Appendix A)

Choose the correct match.

_____ 15.1 Separation of the iris into two layers	A. Blepharoptosis
_____ 15.2 Incision into the bone surrounding the eye	B. Iridocyclochoroiditis
_____ 15.3 Inflamed ciliary body and cornea	C. Orbitotomy
_____ 15.4 Hardening of the lens	D. Iridotasis
_____ 15.5 Softening of the cornea	E. Lacrimotomy
_____ 15.6 Inflammation of the iris, the ciliary body and the choroid	F. Cyclokeratitis
_____ 15.7 Swelling of the eyelid	G. Blepharedema
_____ 15.8 Incision into the tear duct	H. Phacosclerosis
_____ 15.9 Stretching of the iris	I. Keratomalacia
_____ 15.10 Drooping eyelids	J. Iridoschisis

You've got this! Use your new knowledge to decipher these words.

_____ 15.11 Keratoscleritis	A. Inflammation of the cornea and sclera
_____ 15.12 Keratoconjunctivitis	B. Pain of the cornea
_____ 15.13 Iridalgia	C. Softening of the iris
_____ 15.14 Keratalgia	D. Pain in the iris
_____ 15.15 Iridomalacia	E. Inflammation of the sclera and cornea
_____ 15.16 Iridocele	F. Inflammation of the sclera and choroid
_____ 15.17 Sclerochoroiditis	G. Inflammation of the cornea and the conjunctiva
_____ 15.18 Sclerokeratitis	H. A swelling of the iris

Write-in the correct word from the list below.

15.19 Abnormal mobility of the lens _____

15.20 Disease of the choroid _____

15.21 A condition where the
        iris drops out of its position _____

15.22 Incision into the corner of the eye _____

15.23 Removal of corneal tissue/replacement
        with corneal tissue lenticule _____

15.24 Softening of the white of the eye _____

15.25 The removal of the iris
        and the capsule of the lens _____

15.26 Blood in the cornea _____

15.27 Refers to both the orbit and the nose _____

15.28 Inflammation of both
        the choroid and the ciliary body _____

Epikeratophakia	Iridoptosis	Phacoplanesis
Canthotomy	Scleromalacia	Choroidopathy
Orbitonasal	Choroidocyclitis	Iridocapsulectomy
Keratohemia		

Chapter Quiz 2 (Answers in Appendix A)

Choose the correct match.

_____ 15.29 Phacoplanesis	A. The removal of the iris and the capsule of the lens
_____ 15.30 Choroidocyclitis	B. Abnormal mobility of the lens
_____ 15.31 Orbitonasal	C. Softening of the white of the eye
_____ 15.32 Scleromalacia	D. Blood in the cornea
_____ 15.33 Iridocapsulectomy	E. The iris drops out of its position
_____ 15.34 Iridoptosis	F. Removal of corneal tissue/replacement with corneal tissue lenticule
_____ 15.35 Epikeratophakia	G. Inflamed choroid and ciliary body
_____ 15.36 Choroidopathy	H. Incision into the corner of the eye
_____ 15.37 Keratohemia	I. Refers to both the orbit and the nose
_____ 15.38 Canthotomy	J. Disease of the choroid

You've got this! Use your new knowledge to decipher these words.

_____ 15.39 Sclerostomy	A. Inflammation of the sclera, cornea and iris
_____ 15.40 Sclerotomy	B. Inflammation of the iris and choroid
_____ 15.41 Scleroiritis	C. Inflammation of the cornea
_____ 15.42 Sclerokeratoiritis	D. Surgical formation of an opening in the sclera
_____ 15.43 Phakitis	E. Incision of the sclera
_____ 15.44 Cyclitis	F. Inflammation of the sclera and iris
_____ 15.45 Keratoiditis	G. Inflammation of the lens of the eye
_____ 15.46 Iridochorioiditis	H. Inflammation of the ciliary body

Write-in the correct word from the list below.

15.47 Stretching of the iris _____

15.48 Inflammation of the ciliary body and cornea _____

15.49 Drooping eyelids _____

15.50 Softening of the cornea _____

15.51 Incision into the tear duct _____

15.52 Incision into the bone surrounding the eye _____

15.53 Separation of the iris into two layers _____

15.54 Swelling of the eyelid _____

15.55 Inflammation of the iris,
        the ciliary body and the choroid _____

15.56 Hardening of the lens _____

Cyclokeratitis	Blepharedema	Iridotasis
Orbitotomy	Iridoschisis	Keratomalacia
Blepharoptosis	Iridocyclochoroiditis	Phacosclerosis
Lacrimotomy		

Word Tour 3

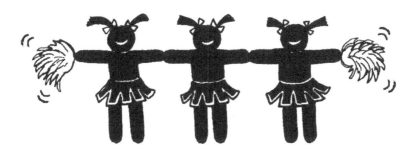

Congratulations! You've made it to the third review. You should be proud of yourself! Take a moment to relax and pat yourself on the back.

Then, when you're ready, forge ahead to these review exercises. Working through these exercises will help you remember the things you've learned so far.

The questions are organized into two parts. You can work them one page at a time and check your answers with each page, or challenge yourself and check your answers after each part.

So, take a moment, then grab your pencil and get started!

NOTES...

Word Tour 3

Part 1 (Answers in Appendix A)

Match the definitions to the terms.

_____ 3.1 Swelling of the eyelid	A. Cyclokeratitis
_____ 3.2 Glaucoma treatment where the iris is stretched	B. Iridotasis
_____ 3.3 Nose bleed	C. Cheilitis
_____ 3.4 Inflammation of the cornea and ciliary body	D. Glossoptosis
_____ 3.5 Condition of having air pockets between the two layers of the pleura	E. Transantral
_____ 3.6 Condition of having calculus in the salivary duct	F. Pneumothorax
_____ 3.7 Reconstruction of the tissue connecting the tongue to the floor of the mouth	G. Sialolithiasis
_____ 3.8 Inflammation of the lip	H. Otosclerosis
_____ 3.9 An approach through a cavity in a bone	I. Epistaxis
_____ 3.10 Hardening of the bones in the ear causing progressive deafness	J. Blepharedema
_____ 3.11 Condition where the position of the tongue drops downward	K. Epiglottis
_____ 3.12 Leaf-shaped covering of the entrance to the larynx	L. Frenoplasty

Write-in the meaning of the term.

3.13 *Naso-* = _____   3.15 *Hypo-* = _____

3.14 *Oro-* = _____   3.16 *Docho-* = _____

Match the definitions to the terms.

_____ 3.17 The outer lobe of the ear

A. Arytenoidectomy

_____ 3.18 A condition where the tissue of the larynx
        softens

B. Iridoschisis

_____ 3.19 Puncture of the chest wall in order to
        remove fluids

C. Thoracentesis

_____ 3.20 Separation of the iris into two layers

D. Palatoglossal

_____ 3.21 Removal of part of the bone that contains
        the sockets for the teeth

E. Labyrinthitis

_____ 3.22 Incision into the corner of the eye

F. Alveolectomy

_____ 3.23 Removal of part of the gum tissue

G. Laryngomalacia

_____ 3.24 Infection of the inner ear

H. Gingivectomy

_____ 3.25 Excision of a laryngeal cartilage

I. Pinna

_____ 3.26 Surgery that binds the two layers of the
        pleura together

J. Canthotomy

_____ 3.27 Concerning the palate and the tongue

K. Myringitis

_____ 3.28 Inflammation of the eardrum

L. Pleurodesis

Write-in the meaning of the term.

3.29 *Tympan-* = _____   3.32 *Myring-* = _____

3.30 *Cheil-* = _____   3.33 *Cantho-* = _____

3.31 *Gloss-* = _____   3.34 *Sialo-* = _____

Match the definitions to the terms.

_____ 3.35 Reconstruction of the ear canal	A. Labioglossolaryngeal
_____ 3.36 Hardening of the lens of the eye	B. Tympanic membrane
_____ 3.37 Infection of a paranasal sinus	C. Ethmoiditis
_____ 3.38 The procedure of taking x-rays of the larynx	D. Laryngography
_____ 3.39 Excision of the border of the lip	E. Lobectomy
_____ 3.40 Softening of the sclera	F. Vermilionectomy
_____ 3.41 Infection of the inner lining of the nose	G. Postauricular
_____ 3.42 Excision of a part of the lung	H. Meatoplasty
_____ 3.43 Eardrum	I. Scleromalacia
_____ 3.44 Concerning the larynx, the lips and the tongue	J. Phacosclerosis
_____ 3.45 Incision into the tear duct	K. Tracheostenosis
_____ 3.46 Behind the outer ear	L. Rhinitis
_____ 3.47 Narrowing of the trachea	M. Lacrimotomy

Write-in the meaning of the term.

3.48 -*malacia* = _____   3.51 -*desis* = _____

3.49 -*edema* = _____   3.52 -*tasis* = _____

3.50 -*pnea* = _____   3.53 -*oxia* = _____

Match the definitions to the terms.

_____ 3.54 Excision of a dead part of the bone | A. Antrotomy

_____ 3.55 Abnormal mobility of the lens | B. Cholesteatoma

_____ 3.56 A fast rate of breathing | C. Keratoiritis

_____ 3.57 Incision into a wall of a bone cavity | D. Sialodochoplasty

_____ 3.58 Reconstructive surgery of a salivary duct | E. Epikeratophakia

_____ 3.59 Puncture of the pleural cavity in order to remove fluids with a needle | F. Pneumopexy

_____ 3.60 Surgical reconstruction involving the lungs and the chest | G. Sublingual

_____ 3.61 Narrowing of the larynx | H. Thoracopneumoplasty

_____ 3.62 Inflammation of the iris and the cornea | I. Laryngostenosis

_____ 3.63 Tumor made of cholesterol and epithelial cells | J. Pleuracentesis

_____ 3.64 Surgical attachment of a lung to the thoracic wall | K. Phacoplanesis

_____ 3.65 Procedure to remove the corneal tissue and replace it with a corneal tissue lenticule | L. Sequestrectomy

_____ 3.66 Below the tongue | M. Tachypnea

Word Tour 3

Part 2 (Answers in Appendix A)

Match the terms to the definitions.

_____ 3.1 Iridotasis	A. Inflammation of the cornea and ciliary body
_____ 3.2 Cyclokeratitis	B. An approach through a cavity in a bone
_____ 3.3 Pneumothorax	C. Glaucoma treatment where the iris is stretched
_____ 3.4 Epistaxis	D. Leaf-shaped covering of the entrance to the larynx
_____ 3.5 Blepharedema	E. Condition of having air pockets between the two layers of the pleura
_____ 3.6 Transantral	F. The outer lobe of the ear
_____ 3.7 Epiglottis	G. A condition where the tissue of the larynx softens
_____ 3.8 Laryngomalacia	H. Hardening of the bones in the ear causing progressive deafness
_____ 3.9 Sialolithiasis	I. Swelling of the eyelid
_____ 3.10 Cheilitis	J. Nose bleed
_____ 3.11 Pinna	K. Inflammation of the lip
_____ 3.12 Otosclerosis	L. Condition of having calculus in the salivary duct

Match the terms to the definitions.

_____ 3.13 Frenoplasty	A. Reconstruction of the tissue connecting the tongue to the floor of the mouth
_____ 3.14 Glossoptosis	B. Removal of part of the bone that contains the sockets for the teeth
_____ 3.15 Alveolectomy	C. Concerning the palate and the tongue
_____ 3.16 Labyrinthitis	D. Incision into the corner of the eye
_____ 3.17 Thoracentesis	E. Surgery that binds the two layers of the pleura together
_____ 3.18 Pleurodesis	F. Separation of the iris into two layers
_____ 3.19 Canthotomy	G. Removal of part of the gum tissue
_____ 3.20 Gingivectomy	H. Excision of a laryngeal cartilage
_____ 3.21 Palatoglossal	I. Infection of the inner ear
_____ 3.22 Iridoschisis	J. Condition where the position of the tongue drops downward
_____ 3.23 Arytenoidectomy	K. Inflammation of the eardrum
_____ 3.24 Myringitis	L. Puncture of the chest wall in order to remove fluids

Write-in the meaning of the term.

3.25 *phak-* = _____   3.28 *Cyan-* = _____

3.26 *Kerato-* = _____   3.29 *Supra-* = _____

3.27 *Post-* = _____   3.30 *Thyro-* = _____

Match the terms to the definitions.

_____ 3.31 Keratomalacia	A. Concerning the larynx, the lips and the tongue
_____ 3.32 Ethmoiditis	B. Softening of the sclera
_____ 3.33 Scleromalacia	C. Incision into a wall of a bone cavity
_____ 3.34 Meatoplasty	D. Infection of the inner lining of the nose
_____ 3.35 Laryngography	E. Excision of a part of the lung
_____ 3.36 Lobectomy	F. The procedure of taking x-rays of the larynx
_____ 3.37 Rhinitis	G. Reconstruction of the ear canal
_____ 3.38 Vermilionectomy	H. Narrowing of the trachea
_____ 3.39 Labioglossolaryngeal	I. Infection of a paranasal sinus
_____ 3.40 Phacoplanesis	J. Softening of the cornea
_____ 3.41 Tracheostenosis	K. Excision of the border of the lip
_____ 3.42 Lacrimotomy	L. Abnormal mobility of the lens
_____ 3.43 Antrotomy	M. Incision into the tear duct

Write-in the meaning of the term.

3.44 *Sub-* = _____

3.45 *Dent-* = _____

3.46 *Labia-* = _____

3.47 *Hemi-* = _____

3.48 *-ptosis* = _____

3.49 *-staxis* = _____

Match the terms to the definitions.

_____ 3.50 Sequestrectomy

_____ 3.51 Tympanic membrane

_____ 3.52 Postauricular

_____ 3.53 Tachypnea

_____ 3.54 Sublingual

_____ 3.55 Epikeratophakia

_____ 3.56 Pneumopexy

_____ 3.57 Pleuracentesis

_____ 3.58 Keratoiritis

_____ 3.59 Sialodochoplasty

_____ 3.60 Laryngostenosis

_____ 3.61 Thoracopneumoplasty

_____ 3.62 Cholesteatoma

A. Surgical attachment of a lung to the thoracic wall

B. Inflammation of the iris and the cornea

C. Tumor made of cholesterol and epithelial cells

D. A fast rate of breathing

E. Narrowing of the larynx

F. Surgical reconstruction involving the lungs and the chest

G. Puncture of the pleural cavity in order to remove fluids with a needle

H. Procedure to remove the corneal tissue and replace it with a corneal tissue lenticule

I. Reconstructive surgery of a salivary duct

J. Below the tongue

K. Eardrum

L. Excision of a dead part of the bone

M. Behind the outer ear

16

The Digestive System, Part 1: The oral cavity and beyond

Let's learn terms that are used with the digestive system. The digestive system has many body parts and organs. As soon as a piece of food touches your lips, it has begun its journey through the digestive system, a journey that takes it through the body organs we'll discuss in this lesson.

It's all GREEK [or Latin] to me!

crico – refers to cartilage in the larynx
-ectasia – to dilate or stretch
esophago – refers to the esophagus
-phagia – eat
xerosis – dryness

16.1
Speaking of lips, we covered the medical terms for lips previously. The patient stayed out in the sun too long and her lips became irritated, or inflamed. What would her doctor call this condition?

_____ Sialitis   _____ Cheilitis   _____ Glossitis

16.2
When we studied the oral cavity you also learned about the salivary glands. What does the doctor call an inflamed salivary gland?

_____ Sialitis   _____ Cheilitis   _____ Glossitis

16.3
Before we explore further than the oral cavity. Do you remember what an inflamed tongue is called?

_____ Sialitis   _____ Cheilitis   _____ Glossitis

16.1

<u>Cheilitis</u> is the inflammation of the lips.

Cheil- is the Greek word for lips. And *-itis* means inflammation.

16.2

The inflammation of the salivary glands is <u>sialitis</u>.

Sial- is from the Greek word for saliva. *Sial- + -itis* is the inflammation of the salivary glands.

16.3

<u>Glossitis</u> is an inflammation of the tongue.

Gloss- is from the Greek word for tongue and *-itis* means inflammation.

QUICK QUIZ *(Answers in Appendix A)*

_____ 16.1 *-ptosis*	**A.** Stretching	
_____ 16.2 *-tasis*	**B.** Lens shaped	
_____ 16.3 *Scler-*	**C.** To drop, to move downward in position	
_____ 16.4 Lenticule	**D.** Refers to the sclera	
_____ 16.5 *Phak-*	**A.** Refers to the lens	
_____ 16.6 *Kerato-*	**B.** Refers to the cornea	
_____ 16.7 *Cyclo-*	**C.** Refers to the ciliary body	
_____ 16.8 *Irido-*	**D.** Refers to the iris	

Quick Review

Meato- = opening or passageway   *Tympano-* = tympanic membrane
Myringa- = like *tympano-*, it means tympanic membrane or eardrum

16.4

As we begin to descend from the mouth, through the digestive system, we enter a passageway called the pharynx. This passageway carries food out of the mouth deeper into the digestive system. Dr. Sharp's patient has a dryness of the pharynx. What is the name of this condition?

_____ Pharyngoparalysis   _____ Pharyngoxerosis   _____ Pharyngodynia

16.5

The pharynx has 3 parts. Which part is behind the mouth?

_____ Nasopharynx   _____ Oropharynx   _____ Laryngopharynx

16.6

Dr. Sharp saw a patient the other day who had a sore throat. What was his diagnosis?

_____ Sialitis   _____ Pharyngoparalysis   _____ Pharyngitis

16.7

Let's say you just took a bite of apple. As you swallow, it goes through the pharynx and enters a longer tube that leads to the stomach, the esophagus. In performing an operation, Dr. Sharp must dilate or stretch the patient's esophagus. This is called:

_____ Esophagectomy   _____ Esophagotomy   _____ Esophagectasia

16.8

Sonny, a two year old, swallowed a paper clip. It's lodged in the esophagus. Dr. Sharp makes an incision into the esophagus to remove it. Which procedure did he perform?

_____ Esophagectomy   _____ Esophagotomy   _____ Esophagostomy

16.9

Dr. Sharp's patient has difficulty swallowing. What is the name of this problem?

_____ Dysphagia   _____ Dyspepsia   _____ Dysmenorrhea

16.4

Pharyngoxerosis is dryness of the pharynx.

Pharyngo- comes from the Greek word for throat. *-xerosis* means dryness. The pharynx also is part of the respiratory system; it transports air to the larynx.

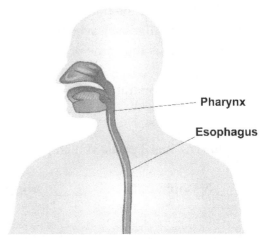

Pharynx

Esophagus

16.5

The oropharynx is behind the mouth.

The nasopharynx is above the palate at the back of the nasal cavity. The oropharynx is at the back of the oral cavity, the mouth. The laryngopharynx is in back of the larynx and leads deeper into the digestive system. Remember the pharynx from The Respiratory System chapter? It's part of both the respiratory and digestive systems.

16.6

A sore throat is pharyngitis.

Pharyng- is from the Greek word for throat. *-itis* is the suffix for inflammation.

16.7

Dilating or stretching the esophagus is esophagectasia.

Esophago- refers to the esophagus and *-ectasia* means to dilate or stretch.

16.8

An esophagotomy is an incision into the esophagus.

Break this word into its parts: *esophago-* is the esophagus; *-tomy* means incision.

16.9

Dysphagia is the inability to swallow.

Dysphagia is composed of two major parts: *dys-* meaning "bad," and *-phagia,* meaning "eat." Notice esophagus has "phag" inside of it.

Dyspepsia, remember, is also related to digestion. It means painful digestion; it's connected with an upset stomach. *Dys-* = bad and *–pepsia* = digestion.

16.10

One condition that causes dysphagia is when a muscle of the cricoid tissue, where the larynx and esophagus join, does not relax and food cannot easily slide into the esophagus. What is the name of this condition?

_____ Cricopharyngeal   _____ Cricotracheotomy   _____ Pharyngolith
          achalasia

16.11

To correct the cricopharyngeal achalasia, Dr. Sharp performed a myotomy. What did Dr. Sharp do?

_____ removed the esophagus

_____ made an incision into the muscle of the cricoid tissue, pharynx and
          esophagus

_____ sutured the cricoid cartilage and the pharynx muscle

16.12

A sphincter is a muscle ring that can open and close a passage. Dr. Sharp sees another patient with achalasia. Her cardiac sphincter is not relaxing and food can not move from the esophagus into the stomach. Where is the cardiac sphincter located?

_____ Top of   _____ Middle of   _____ Bottom of
          esophagus   esophagus   esophagus

16.13

To correct the patient's achalasia, Dr. Sharp dilates or widens the sphincter by placing a balloon inside and inflating it. He uses an instrument that allows him to see into the esophagus and place the balloon. What procedure did he perform?

_____ Esophagotomy   _____ Esophagoscopy   _____ Esophagostomy

16.14

You've got this! Let's see how much word power you've developed. What is the meaning of esophagectomy?

_____

16.10

<u>Cricopharyngeal achalasia</u> is the name of the condition.

Crico- is cartilage in the larynx; *-pharyngeal* refers to the pharynx tissue. Achalasia means failure to relax. In this condition, this muscle ring, the cricopharyngeal ring, is so tight that food cannot easily slide into the esophagus.

16.11

Dr. Sharp performed an <u>incision into the muscle tissue of the cricoid cartilage, the pharynx, and the esophagus.</u>

Myotomy is an incision into the muscle. *Myo-* means muscle; *-tomy* means incision.

16.12

The cardiac sphincter is at the <u>bottom of the esophagus.</u>

The cardiac sphincter is the name of the muscle ring that joins the esophagus with the stomach. When it relaxes, the food continues its journey into the stomach. If it cannot relax, the food or some portion of it is blocked in the esophagus.

16.13

The procedure of looking inside the esophagus is an <u>esophagoscopy.</u>

esophago- means esophagus; and *-scopy* means to look. The doctor is using an esophagoscope to look into the esophagus. Attached to the scope is a balloon that the doctor places inside the muscle ring and inflates.

16.14

Esophagectomy is the <u>removal of a section of the esophagus.</u>

esophag- means esophagus; and *-ectomy* means surgical removal.

Here's a few more terms we will practice.

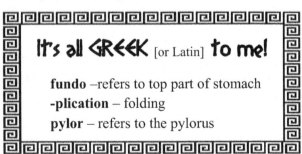

It's all GREEK [or Latin] to me!

fundo –refers to top part of stomach
-plication – folding
pylor – refers to the pylorus

16.15

Since Dr. Sharp removed the bottom part of the esophagus, he had to create a new opening between the esophagus and the stomach. What is this procedure?

_____ Pharyngogastrostomy   _____ Esophagogastrostomy
_____ Pyloroplasty

16.16

Dr. Sharp's patient has pain in the area around the sphincter between the stomach and intestines. What is the name of this condition?

_____ Pyloristenosis   _____ Pyloralgia   _____ Proctalgia

16.17

Dr. Sharp discovers that the patient has pain in the area around the sphincter between the stomach and the intestines because of constriction and narrowing of this area. What is the name of this condition?

_____ Pyloristenosis   _____ Pyloralgia   _____ Proctalgia

16.18

Mike has an ulcer. Dr. Sharp operates, opening and widening the pylorus. What is this procedure?

_____ Pylorogastrectomy   _____ Pylorospasm   _____ Pyloroplasty

16.19

The lower half of the stomach is called the antrum. If a patient has a persistent perforating ulcer, the doctor may remove the antrum and the pylorus. Which procedure does NOT describe this operation?

_____ Antrectomy   _____ Hemigastrectomy   _____ Pylorotomy

16.15
Esophagogastrostomy is an opening between the esophagus and the stomach.

This word has three major parts: *esophago-* which stands for the esophagus; *gastro-* which stands for the stomach; and *-stomy* which stands for the opening created between them in order to rejoin them after part of the esophagus was removed.

16.16
Pyloralgia is pain in the area of the pylorus - the narrow passage connecting the stomach to the small intestines (the pyloric sphincter).

Pylor- refers to the pylorus and *–algia* means pain.

16.17
Constriction of the pylorus is pyloristenosis.

Pylor- refers to the pylorus and *–stenosis* means constriction or narrowing.

16.18
Pyloroplasty is reconstruction of the pylorus.

This word is made of two major parts: *pyloro-* refers to the pylorus; *-plasty* refers to an operation that repairs or reforms an organ or body part.

A pyloroplasty is usually performed to stretch the opening inside the pylorus.

16.19
Pylorotomy does not describe the operation of removing the antrum and the pylorus. Remember, *-tomy* means incision into, not removal of.

Pylorotomy is made of two word parts: *pylor-* refers to the pylorus; and *-tomy* refers to a surgical incision. This operation is the surgical incision into the pylorus. Dr. Sharp did more than an incision; he removed the lower part of the stomach: antrectomy or hemigastrectomy are the terms that describe this operation. Antrum is the bottom half of the stomach. An antrectomy is the removal of the bottom half of the stomach. *Antr-* refers to the antrum and *–ectomy* means excision or removal. Hemigastrectomy means the same thing. *Hemi-* means half, *gastr-* means stomach and *–ectomy* means excision.

16.20

Dr. Sharp also performs a vagotomy for his patient with the duodenal ulcer. What did he do?

_____ Cut a small segment of the vagus nerve trunk
_____ Removed the vagus nerve trunk
_____ Sutured the vagus nerve trunk; it was cut during the antrectomy

16.21

The upper part of the stomach is the fundus. Dr. Sharp reduces the size of the opening into the fundus of the stomach for achalasia patients to reduce the chance of food returning to the esophagus. What is this procedure?

_____ Fundusectomy   _____ Fundoscopy   _____ Fundoplication

16.22

One of Dr. Sharp's patient's has a hiatal hernia. Dr. Sharp performs a type of fundoplication. He wraps part of the fundus around the esophagus, and sutures it in place. This keeps the stomach from going up into the chest. What is this procedure?

_____ Esophagogastric fundoplasty   _____ Esophagostomy
_____ Gastrostomy

16.23

Dr. Sharp performed a surgery where he made a connection between the throat and the stomach. What is this procedure called?

_____ Hemigastrectomy
_____ Esophagostomy
_____ Pharyngogastrostomy

16.24

You've got this! Let's see how much word power you've developed. Here's a term we haven't shown you yet, but you'll be able to decipher its meaning. What is the meaning of pharyngoscopy?

_____

16.20

During a vagotomy the doctor <u>cuts a small segment of the vagus nerve trunk</u>.

Vag- refers to the vagus nerve and *–tomy* means incision or cut.

16.21

<u>Fundoplication</u> is the surgical reduction of the size of the opening into the stomach.

Fundo- refers to the top part of the stomach where the esophagus and the stomach meet. *–plication* refers to folding. Fundoplasty may also describe this procedure. *–plasty* means to repair or reconstruct.

16.22

<u>Esophagogastric fundoplasty</u> reforms the fundus of the stomach, and the esophagus is involved in the repair.

Esophagogastric is a long word with two major parts: *esophago-* refers to the esophagus; *-gastric* refers to the stomach. Look at fundoplasty: *fundo-* refers to the fundus and *-plasty* means to repair.

16.23

<u>Pharyngogastrostomy</u> is the surgical connection of the throat and the stomach.

Pharyngo- refers to the pharynx or throat. *Gastro-* refers to the stomach. *–stomy* is a surgical connection.

16.24

Pharyngoscopy is a <u>visual exam of the throat.</u>

Pharyngo- refers to the throat. *–scopy* is a visual exam using an instrument.

QUICK QUIZ *(Answers in Appendix A)*

_____ 16.13 *-phagia*	**A.** To eat
_____ 16.14 Achalasia	**B.** Cartilage in the larynx
_____ 16.15 *Crico-*	**C.** Refers to the esophagus
_____ 16.16 *Esophago-*	**D.** Failure to relax

Chapter Quiz 1 (Answers in Appendix A)

Choose the correct match.

_____ 16.1 Uppermost part of stomach	A. Pharynx
_____ 16.2 Surgical incision through vagus nerve	B. Fundus
_____ 16.3 Repair of the part of the stomach that opens into the duodenum	C. Vagotomy
_____ 16.4 Tube between the pharynx and stomach	D. Pharyngogastrostomy
_____ 16.5 The throat	E. Pyloroplasty
_____ 16.6 Inability to swallow	F. Dysphagia
_____ 16.7 Inability of the muscle to relax	G. Fundoplication
_____ 16.8 Muscle ring between the esophagus and the stomach	H. Cardiac sphincter
_____ 16.9 Surgical connection of the throat and the stomach	I. Esophagus
_____ 16.10 Surgical reduction of the size of the opening into the stomach	J. Achalasia

You've got this! Use your new knowledge to decipher these words.

_____ 16.11 Hemiglossectomy	A. Surgical removal of half of the liver
_____ 16.12 Hemihepatectomy	B. Repair of the esophagus and stomach
_____ 16.13 Pyloristenosis	C. Pain around the pylorus
_____ 16.14 Pyloralgia	D. Narrowing of the esophagus
_____ 16.15 Esophagocele	E. Softening of the esophageal walls
_____ 16.16 Esophagomalacia	F. Swelling of the esophagus
_____ 16.17 Esophagostenosis	G. Narrowing of the pylorus
_____ 16.18 Esophagogastroplasty	H. Surgical removal of half of the tongue

Write-in the correct word from the list below.

16.19 Removal of the bottom
        part of the stomach _____

16.20 Reforms the upper part of
        the stomach around the esophagus _____

16.21 Inflammation of the lips _____

16.22 Inflammation of the salivary glands _____

16.23 Inflammation of the tongue _____

16.24 Visual examination of the throat _____

16.25 The back of the oral cavity _____

16.26 Inflammation of the throat - a sore throat _____

16.27 Visual exam of the tube between
        the pharynx and stomach _____

16.28 Above the palate at the back of the nasal cavity _____

Cheilitis	Sialitis	Nasopharynx
Esophagoscopy	Oropharynx	Pharyngoscopy
Pharyngitis	Antrectomy	Fundoplasty
Glossitis		

Chapter Quiz 2 (Answers in Appendix A)

Choose the correct match.

_____ 16.29 Pharyngoscopy	A. Inflammation of the tongue
_____ 16.30 Esophagoscopy	B. Visual exam of the tube between the pharynx and the stomach
_____ 16.31 Cheilitis	C. Inflammation of the throat - a sore throat
_____ 16.32 Antrectomy	D. Above the palate at the back of the nasal cavity
_____ 16.33 Sialitis	E. Reforms the upper part of stomach around the esophagus
_____ 16.34 Oropharynx	F. Inflammation of the lips
_____ 16.35 Pharyngitis	G. Inflammation of the salivary glands
_____ 16.36 Fundoplasty	H. Removal of the bottom part of the stomach
_____ 16.37 Glossitis	I. Visual examination of the throat
_____ 16.38 Nasopharynx	J. The back of the oral cavity

You've got this! Use your new knowledge to decipher these words.

_____ 16.39 Esophagogastro-anastomosis	A. Making a connection between the esophagus and intestine
_____ 16.40 Esophagostomy	B. Inflamed condition of the pylorus
_____ 16.41 Esophagoptosis	C. Excision of the cricoid cartilage
_____ 16.42 Esophagoenterostomy	D. Joining the esophagus to the stomach
_____ 16.43 Cricoidectomy	E. Refers to one-half of the chest
_____ 16.44 Pylorectomy	F. Dropping of the esophagus
_____ 16.45 Pyloritis	G. Surgical removal of the pylorus
_____ 16.46 Hemithorax	H. Surgical formation of an opening into the esophagus

Write-in the correct word from the list below.

16.47 Surgical reduction of the size
of the opening into the stomach _____

16.48 Surgical connection of the throat and the stomach _____

16.49 The throat _____

16.50 Surgical incision through vagus nerve _____

16.51 Inability to swallow _____

16.52 Uppermost part of stomach _____

16.53 Repair of the part of the stomach
that opens into the duodenum _____

16.54 Tube between pharynx and stomach _____

16.55 Inability of the muscle to relax _____

16.56 Muscle ring between
the esophagus and the stomach _____

Pharynx	Cardiac sphincter	Pyloroplasty
Dysphagia	Fundus	Achalasia
Esophagus	Pharyngogastrostomy	Vagotomy
Fundoplication		

17

The Digestive System, Part 2: Easy to digest, honest

In this chapter we will cover a few more terms and get lots more practice.

17.1

Dr. Sharp's patient had a peptic ulcer. Dr. Sharp did tests to determine the cause. He found the cause was a chronic inflammation of the gall bladder. What is the name of this condition?

_____ Cholecystalgia
_____ Cholecystitis
_____ Cholecystogram

CLUE

The key is the suffix! "Inflammation" appears right on page 1 of this book!

17.2

The gallbladder has two major parts: the bladder and the ducts. Its ducts connect it to the liver and the duodenum. Which disease below refers to an inflammatory problem in the duct?

_____ Cholecystalgia   _____ Cholangiolitis   _____ Cholecystogram

17.3

What if Dr. Sharp's patient has an inflammation of the common bile duct, the big one? This duct is used by the pancreas, the liver, and the gallbladder. What's the name of this disease?

_____ Cholecystogram   _____ Cholangitis   _____ Choledochitis

17.1
<u>Cholecystitis</u> is the inflammation of the bladder that stores bile, or the gallbladder.

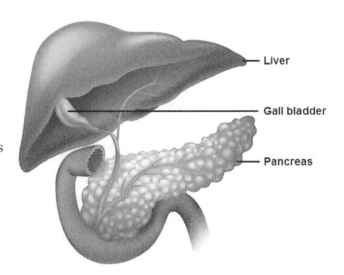

chole- refers to bile; *cyst -* refers to the bladder; and *-itis* refers to inflammation.

17.2
<u>Cholangiolitis</u> is inflammation of the gall bladder duct.

Cholangiolitis has three major word parts: *chol-* refers to bile; *angio-* refers to vessel; *-itis* refers to inflammation. Remember, you've seen the word part, *angio-*, before. Angiitis is the inflammation of a blood or lymph vessel. In this word, the vessel is the smaller bile ducts.

17.3
<u>Choledochitis</u> is inflammation of the common bile duct.

Choledochitis has three major word parts: *chole-* refers to bile; *doch-* refers to duct; and *-itis* refers to inflammation. When *doch-* is combined with *chole-*, it always refers to the largest duct, the common bile duct.

QUICK QUIZ *(Answers in Appendix A)*

_____ 17.1 *Oto-*	**A.** Colon
_____ 17.2 *Colo-*	**B.** Uterus or womb
_____ 17.3 *Cephalo-*	**C.** Ear
_____ 17.4 *Hystero-*	**D.** Head

_____ 17.5 *-stomy*	**A.** A surgical removal
_____ 17.6 *-ectomy*	**B.** A surgical reconstruction
_____ 17.7 *-tomy*	**C.** A surgical opening
_____ 17.8 *-plasty*	**D.** A surgical incision

17.4

Dr. Sharp's patient has a peptic ulcer. He suspects the gallbladder is inflamed. He x-rays the gallbladder. What is the result of the x-ray called?

_____ Cholecystogram   _____ Cholangiography   _____ Choledochography

17.5

Dr. Sharp's patient has a stone in the gall bladder. What's the name of this disease?

_____ Cholecystolithiasis
_____ Cholangioma
_____ Choledocholithiasis

CLUE

The key term here is the term for bladder!

17.6

Dr. Sharp has to suture the end of the common bile duct after an operation. What's the name of this procedure?

_____ Cholecystolithotripsy   _____ Cholangiography
_____ Choledochorrhaphy

17.7

Dr. Sharp's patient has a problem with the gallbladder. It has dropped downward. Dr. Sharp sutures it to the abdomen wall to fix it in its proper place. What's the name of this procedure?

_____ Choledochoplasty   _____ Cholecystopexy   _____ Choleangiostomy

17.8

What's another name for the gallbladder and its ducts?

_____ Biliary tract   _____ Gallstone   _____ Pancreas

17.9

Dr. Sharp has to remove the common bile duct. Next, he will connect the gall bladder with the small intestines. What is the name of the procedure to remove the duct?

CLUE

The medical term for duct sounds a lot like its Latin origin!

_____ Cholecystectomy
_____ Choledochectomy   _____ Cholangiectasis

17.4
Cholecystogram is the result of an x-ray of the gallbladder.

Cholecystogram has three major word parts: *chole-* refers to bile; *cyst-* refers to the bladder; and *-gram* is the results of the x-ray. Notice the other word choices indicate that the doctor is taking x-rays of the small ducts and the common bile duct. *-graphy* is the suffix for the examination; *-gram* is the suffix for the results of that examination, the actual x-ray that the doctor looks at.

17.5
A patient may have a gallstone in the gall bladder; that's called cholecystolithiasis.

Cholecystolithiasis has four major word parts: *chole-* refers to bile; *cysto-* refers to bladder; *lith-* refers to stones and *-iasis* means disease.

17.6
Choledochorrhaphy is suturing the common bile duct.

Choledochorrhaphy has three major word parts: *chole-* refers to bile; *docho-* refers to the common bile duct; and *-rrhaphy* refers to suturing.

17.7
Cholecystopexy is the fixation of the gallbladder to the abdomen wall.

Cholecystopexy has three major parts: *chole-* refers to bile; *cysto-* refers to the bladder; *-pexy* means to affix something so it is tightly held.

17.8
The biliary tract is another word for the organs and ducts that are involved in the secretion, storage, and delivery of bile to the duodenum.

The biliary tract includes the gallbladder, its ducts, and sometimes the liver. Notice the similarity between "bile" and "biliary"?

17.9
Choledochectomy is the surgical removal of part of the common bile duct.

Choledochectomy has three major word parts: *chole-* stands for bile; *doch-* stands for the common bile duct; and *-ectomy* stands for surgical removal.

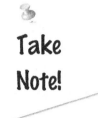

Take Note!   *Remember, when you see "doch" in a word that starts with "chole," it refers to the common bile duct.*

17.10
Now Dr. Sharp has to connect the gall bladder with the small intestines. What is the name of this procedure?

_____ Cholangiogastrostomy   _____ Cholecystnephrostomy
_____ Cholecystenterostomy

17.11
The patient has a stone in the pancreas. What is the name of the procedure used to remove the stone?

_____ Pancreatectomy   _____ Pancreatotomy   _____ Pancreatolithectomy

17.12
Dr. Sharp's patient had an infection of the pancreas. What is the name of this condition?

_____ Pancreatectomy   _____ Pancreatitis   _____ Pancreatorrhaphy

17.13
Dr. Sharp has to create an artificial opening between the pancreas and the small intestines. What is the name of this procedure?

_____ Pancreaticocholecystostomy   _____ Pancreatogastrostomy
_____ Pancreatoduodenostomy

17.14
You've got this! Let's see how much word power you've developed. What is the meaning of cholangiopancreatography?

_____

17.10
Cholecystenterostomy is the surgical connection of the gallbladder and the small intestine.

Cholecystenterostomy consists of four major parts: *chole-* refers to bile; *cyst-* refers to bladder, *entero-* refers to the small intestines, and *-stomy* refers to the surgical connection of these two body parts.

17.11
Pancreatolithectomy is the procedure to remove stones from the pancreas.

Pancreato- refers to the pancreas, *lith-* means stone and *–ectomy* means surgical removal. The pancreas excretes juices to the small intestine to help with digestion.

17.12
Pancreatitis is the inflammation of the pancreas.

Pancreatitis is composed of two major word parts: *pancreat-* refers to the pancreas; *-itis* refers to inflammation.

17.13
Pancreatoduodenostomy is an artificial opening between the pancreas and the small intestines.

This word is made of three major parts: *pancreato-* refers to the pancreas; *duodeno-* refers to the duodenum, a part of the small intestines; and *-stomy* refers to a surgical opening between two body organs or body parts. Remember, the duodenum? It's the first part of the intestines. It joins the stomach at the pyloric sphincter.

17.14
Cholangiopancreatography is taking an x-ray of the gall bladder ducts and the pancreas.

Cholangiopancreatography has three major word parts: *cholang-* refers to the gall bladder ducts; *pancreato-* refers to the pancreas; and *-graphy* refers to the examination using an x-ray machine or other method of "seeing" the inside organs.

17.15

Dr. Sharp found stones in his patient's common duct. Now he has to connect the duct to the small intestine for drainage. What's this procedure called?

_____ Cholecystenterostomy
_____ Choledochoduodenostomy
_____ Choledocholithiasis

CLUE

The parts are: bile > duct > duodenum > surgical opening!

17.16

Dr. Sharp's patient has a tumor in the common duct. After removing that part of the duct, and part of the duodenum, Dr. Sharp connects the remaining part of the duct to the second part of the small intestines. What's this procedure called?

_____ Choledochojejunostomy   _____ Hepaticojejunostomy
_____ Cholecystenterostomy

17.17

This patient has a tumor where the common duct and the liver meet. After removing the tumor, Dr. Sharp connects the liver to the jejunum. What's the name of this operation?

_____ Choledochojejunostomy   _____ Hepaticojejunostomy
_____ Gastrojejunostomy

17.18

Dr. Sharp's patient has a pancreatic pseudocyst. To treat the cyst, Dr. Sharp drains it by surgically connecting it to the stomach. What's the name of this procedure?

_____ Cystoduodenostomy   _____ Cystojejunostomy
_____ Cystogastrostomy

17.19

Dr. Sharp's patient has an adenocarcinoma in the pancreas. Dr. Sharp removes the pancreas and the first part of the small intestines. What's the name of the operation?

_____ Pancreatoduodenostomy   _____ Pancreatoduodenectomy
_____ Pancreaticojejunostomy

17.15
Choledochoduodenostomy is the surgical connection of the common bile duct to the small intestine.

Choledochoduodenostomy is made of 4 major parts: *chole-* refers to bile; *docho-* refers to the common duct; *duodeno-* refers to the duodenum, the part of the intestines that connects to the stomach; and *-stomy* refers to a surgical opening made in the body in order to connect it to another body organ or part.

17.16
Choledochojejunostomy is the surgical joining of the common bile duct to the jejunum of the small intestine

Choledochojejunostomy is composed of four major parts: *chole-* refers to bile; *docho-* refers to the common duct; *jejuno-* refers to the second part of the small intestines; and *-stomy* refers to the surgical joining of two body parts by creating an opening between them.

17.17
Hepaticojejunostomy is the surgical connection of the liver to the jejunum.

This word is composed of three major parts: *hepatico-* refers to liver; *jejuno-* refers to the jejunum, a part of the small intestines; *-ostomy* refers to the surgical opening between two body parts.

17.18
Cystogastrostomy is the surgical connection of a cyst, usually in the pancreas, to the stomach.

Cystogastrostomy has three major parts: *cysto-* refers to cyst; *gastro-* refers to stomach; *-stomy* refers to the surgical operation that joins these two parts by making an opening between them and suturing them together.

17.19
Pancreatoduodenectomy is the removal of the pancreas and the first part of the small intestines.

This word has three major parts: *pancreato-* refers to the pancreas; *duoden-* refers to the duodenum, the first part of the small intestine; and *-ectomy* refers to the surgical removal of a body part.

Here's a couple of more terms to
add to your vocabulary.

It's all GREEK [or Latin] to me!

laparo – refers to the abdomen
sigmoido – refers to part of the colon

17.20
Dr. Sharp has a patient whose small intestine is obstructed. Dr. Sharp makes an
incision into the small intestine so he can insert a tube for decompression. What's
this operation?

_____ Enterolysis   _____ Enterotomy   _____ Colotomy

17.21
The next patient also has an obstruction in the intestines. Nothing passes beyond
the obstruction. Dr. Sharp explores the intestines, finding adhesive bands binding
the passage. He frees the intestines. What's this operation?

_____ Enterolysis   _____ Enterotomy   _____ Colotomy

17.22
Dr. Sharp's patient has Crohn's disease in the small bowel. He has to operate
because of a tear. He removes a small part of the bowel and connects the two ends
created by the surgery. What's the name of this operation?

_____ Ileoileostomy   _____ Duodenotomy   _____ Colostomy

17.23

CLUE

Dr. Sharp's patient has an inflammation
that is affecting both the small and large
intestines. What's this disease?

*See the
Greek/Latin box
on page 261!*

_____ Colitis   _____ Duodenitis   _____ Ileocolitis

17.24
Dr. Sharp wants to examine the inside of the large intestines to look for polyps.
What's this procedure?

_____ Colonorrhagia   _____ Colonoscopy   _____ Colostomy

17.20

Enterotomy is a surgical incision into the small intestines.

Enterotomy is composed of two major word parts: *entero-* refers to the intestines and *-tomy* refers to a surgical incision.

17.21

Enterolysis is the freeing of adhesions in the intestines.

Enterolysis is made up of two major word parts: *entero-* refers to the intestines and *-lysis* refers to the dissolution of adhesions.

17.22

Ileoileostomy is connecting two parts of the ileum together.

This word is made of two major word parts: *ileo-* refers to the third part of the small intestines; *-ostomy* refers to the surgical creation of a connection between these two parts. *Ileo-* is used twice to indicate that the surgical connection was between two separate parts of that body part, in this case the ileum.

17.23

Ileocolitis is an inflammation that is affecting both the small and large intestines.

This word is made of three major word parts: *ileo-* refers to the third part of the small intestines; *col-* refers to the large intestines; *-itis* refers to inflammation.

17.24

Colonoscopy is a visual exam of the large intestines, the colon.

This word is made of two major word parts: *colono-*refers to the colon or the large intestines; and *-scopy* refers to the scope, or instrument, used to visually examine the inside of a body part.

QUICK QUIZ *(Answers in Appendix A)*

_____ 17.9 *-pexy*	**A.** Duct
_____ 17.10 *Chole-*	**B.** Bladder
_____ 17.11 *Doch-*	**C.** To affix
_____ 17.12 *Cyst-*	**D.** Bile

QUICK QUIZ *(Answers in Appendix A)*

_____ 17.13 *-malacia*	**A.** Breath
_____ 17.14 *-edema*	**B.** Softness
_____ 17.15 *-pnea*	**C.** Binding
_____ 17.16 *-desis*	**D.** Swelling

_____ 17.17 Thoracostomy	**A.** The condition of blood accumulated in the pleural space
_____ 17.18 Hemothorax	**B.** Binding the two layers of the pleura together
_____ 17.19 Thoracentesis	**C.** Creating an opening into the chest
_____ 17.20 Pleurodesis	**D.** Using a needle to puncture the chest wall

17.25

Often times when Dr. Sharp performs surgery on the digestive tract, he uses a scope and enters through the abdomen. What kind of procedure is this?

_____ Proctoscopy   _____ Laparoscopy   _____ Colonoscopy

17.26

Dr. Sharp's patient has cancer in the descending colon. The doctor removes the affected part of the colon and reconnects it to the rectum. What's this procedure?

_____ Sigmoidoproctostomy   _____ Proctoplasty   _____ Colostomy

17.27

You've got this! Let's see how much word power you've developed. Here's a medical term we haven't shown you yet, but you'll be able to decipher its meaning. What is the meaning of colonorrhagia?

_____

17.25

Laparoscopy is the visual exam of the abdomen.

This word is made of two major word parts: *laparo-* refers to the abdomen; *-scopy* refers to a procedure during which the doctor uses an instrument that allows the doctor to see inside the body.

17.26

Sigmoidoproctostomy is connecting the sigmoid portion of the colon with the rectum.

sigmoido- refers to the lower part of the descending colon; *procto-* refers to the rectum, the part of the intestines right below the sigmoid segment; and *-stomy* refers to the surgical connection of these two parts of the intestines.

17.27

Colonorrhagia is hemorrhaging from the colon.

This word is made of two major word parts: *colono-* refers to the colon or the large intestines; and *-rrhagia* refers to hemorrhaging, or losing a lot of blood.

QUICK QUIZ *(Answers in Appendix A)*

_____ 17.21 Glottis	**A.** Dark blue
_____ 17.22 Cyan	**B.** Two vocal folds and the space that enables us to make sounds
_____ 17.23 Supraglottic	**C.** Below the glottis
_____ 17.24 Subglottis	**D.** Above the glottis

_____ 17.25 Laryngomalacia	**A.** Softening of the larynx tissues
_____ 17.26 Laryngoedema	**B.** Swelling of the larynx
_____ 17.27 Pneumothorax	**C.** A surgically created opening in the trachea
_____ 17.28 Tracheostomy	**D.** The accumulation of air in the chest

_____ 17.29 Cardiovascular	**A.** An opening in the pericardium
_____ 17.30 Pericardium	**B.** The sac enclosing the heart
_____ 17.31 Pericardiostomy	**C.** Inflammation of the pericardium
_____ 17.32 Pericarditis	**D.** Heart and blood vessels

Chapter Quiz 1 (Answers in Appendix A)

Choose the correct match.

_____ 17.1 X-ray showing the gall bladder	A. Choledochoduodenostomy
_____ 17.2 Removal of the common duct of the gall bladder	B. Choledochectomy
_____ 17.3 Visual exam of the abdomen	C. Pancreatoduodenostomy
_____ 17.4 The gall bladder and its ducts	D. Hepaticojejunostomy
_____ 17.5 Surgical connection of small intestines and gall bladder	E. Cholecystogram
_____ 17.6 Surgical connection of common duct and small intestines	F. Laparoscopy
_____ 17.7 X-ray of bile ducts and pancreas	G. Biliary tract
_____ 17.8 Artificial opening between pancreas and small intestines	H. Cholecystenterostomy
_____ 17.9 Surgical connection of the liver and the small intestines	I. Cholangiopancreatography

You've got this! Use your new knowledge to decipher these words.

_____ 17.10 Cholecystnephrostomy	A. Gall stones in the common duct
_____ 17.11 Jejunocolostomy	B. Pain in the gall bladder
_____ 17.12 Choledocholithiasis	C. Surgical connection of the gall bladder and the kidneys
_____ 17.13 Cholecystalgia	D. A tumor of the bile ducts
_____ 17.14 Cholangioma	E. Formation of an artificial passage between the jejunum and colon

Write-in the correct word from the list below.

17.15 Inflammation of the bile ducts _____

17.16 Affixing the gallbladder in place _____

17.17 Removing stones from the pancreas_____

17.18 Inflammation of the gallbladder _____

17.19 Inflammation of the common bile duct _____

17.20 A stone in the gall bladder _____

17.21 Suturing the end of the common bile duct _____

17.22 An infection of the pancreas _____

17.23 Freeing of intestinal adhesions _____

17.24 Inflammation affecting both
        small and large intestines _____

Pancreatolithectomy	Choledochitis	Enterolysis
Cholecystolithiasis	Pancreatitis	Cholecystitis
Choledochorrhaphy	Ileocolitis	Cholangiolitis
Cholecystopexy		

Chapter Quiz 2 (Answers in Appendix A)

Choose the correct match.

_____ 17.25 Enterolysis	A. Inflammation of the common bile duct
_____ 17.26 Cholecystolithiasis	B. Inflammation of the gallbladder
_____ 17.27 Choledocholithiasis	C. Surgical connection of the gall bladder and the kidneys
_____ 17.28 Cholecystitis	D. Visual exam of the abdomen
_____ 17.29 Choledochitis	E. An infection of the pancreas
_____ 17.30 Choledochorrhaphy	F. Gall stones in the common duct
_____ 17.31 Laparoscopy	G. Freeing of intestinal adhesions
_____ 17.32 Cholecystnephrostomy	H. A stone in the gall bladder
_____ 17.33 Pancreatitis	I. Pain in the gall bladder
_____ 17.34 Cholecystalgia	J. Suturing the end of the common bile duct

You've got this! Use your new knowledge to decipher these words.

_____ 17.35 Enterospasm	A. Abnormal enlargement of the intestines
_____ 17.36 Enteroptosis	B. Excision of the gallbladder
_____ 17.37 Enterorrhaphy	C. Painful contractions of the intestines
_____ 17.38 Enteromegaly	D. Forming an opening in the common bile duct
_____ 17.39 Enteropexy	E. Downward drooping of the intestines
_____ 17.40 Cholangiocarcinoma	F. Cancer of the bile ducts
_____ 17.41 Cholecystectomy	G. Suturing of the intestines
_____ 17.42 Choledochostomy	H. Fixation of intestine to abdominal wall

Write-in the correct word from the list below.

17.43 X-ray of the gall bladder _____

17.44 Surgical connection of
        small intestines and gall bladder _____

17.45 Removal of the common duct of the gall bladder _____

17.46 Surgical connection of the
        liver and the small intestines _____

17.47 Surgical connection of
        common duct and small intestines _____

17.48 Inflammation affecting
        both small and large intestines _____

17.49 A tumor of the bile ducts _____

17.50 The gall bladder and its ducts _____

17.51 Artificial opening between
        the pancreas and small intestines _____

17.52 X-ray exam of the bile ducts and the pancreas _____

Cholecystenterostomy	Hepaticojejunostomy	Ileocolitis
Pancreatoduodenostomy	Choledochectomy	Biliary tract
Cholangiopancreatography	Cholecystogram	Cholangioma
Choledochoduodenostomy		

18

The Reproductive System: What's an oo-phor? And other reproductive system terms

Let's look at a few Latin and Greek words that are used when describing diseases and treatment for the reproductive system.

It's all GREEK [or Latin] to me!

cervice – refers to neck of a body part
colp – refers to the vagina
oophor – refers to the ovaries
salping – refers to the ovarian ducts
trachel – refers to neck of a body part

18.1
Here's one you already know. What does *hystero-* refer to?

_____ Ovaries   _____ Womb   _____ Vagina

18.2
Dr. Sharp removes his patient's womb. What's the name of this procedure?

_____ Hysterectomy   _____ Hysterotomy   _____ Hysteroscopy

18.3
Dr. Sharp's next patient's uterus has dropped into her vagina. Dr. Sharp replaces it in its orginal position and affixes it to the vaginal wall. What's this procedure?

_____ Hysterectomy   _____ Hysterotomy   _____ Hysteropexy

18.4
Dr. Sharp must remove the patient's right ovary. What's this procedure?

_____ Salpingopexy   _____ Oophorectomy   _____ Colporrhaphy

18.1

Hystero- refers to the <u>womb</u>.

Hystero- is the Greek word for uterus.

18.2

<u>Hysterectomy</u> is the surgical removal of the womb.

Hystero- refers to womb and *-ectomy* means its surgical removal.

18.3

<u>Hysteropexy</u> is the surgical fixation of the womb.

This word has two major parts: *hystero-* refers to the uterus or womb; *-pexy* refers to the surgical fixation of a body part.

18.4

An <u>oophorectomy</u> is the surgical removal of the ovaries, or of an ovary.

This word is composed of two parts: *oophor-* is a Greek word part meaning to bear eggs; and *-ectomy* means the surgical removal of a body part.

Female Reproductive System

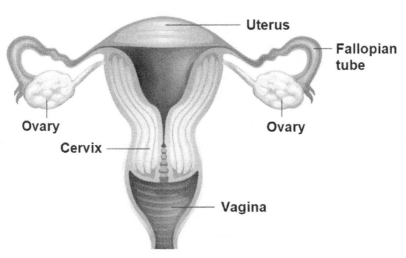

18.5

Dr. Sharp's next patient has a problem with her vagina. Dr. Sharp must remove it. What's the name of this procedure?

_____ Salpingopexy   _____ Oophorectomy   _____ Colpectomy

18.6

Dr. Sharp's next patient has a problem with her ovarian ducts. Dr. Sharp must remove them. What's the name of this procedure?

_____ Salpingectomy   _____ Salpingopexy   _____ Colpectomy

18.7

Dr. Sharp's next patient's vagina has moved out of its normal place. Dr. Sharp replaces it in its original position and fixes it to the abdomen wall. What's the name of this procedure?

_____ Hysteropexy   _____ Colpopexy   _____ Oophoropexy

18.8

Dr. Sharp's next patient's ovarian tube has moved out of its normal place. Dr. Sharp replaces it in its original position and fixes it to the abdomen wall. What's the name of this procedure?

_____ Salpingopexy   _____ Hysteropexy   _____ Oophoropexy

18.9

The ovary of Dr. Sharp's patient has to be affixed to the abdomen wall so that it will remain in its normal position. What's this procedure?

_____ Salpingopexy   _____ Colpopexy   _____ Oophoropexy

18.10

Dr. Sharp orders a hysterosalpingography. What does he want to look at?

_____ the womb and the ovary
_____ the womb and the ovary duct
_____ the vagina and the ovary

18.5
Colpectomy is the surgical removal of the vagina.

This word is composed of two parts: *colp-* is from the Greek word meaning vagina; *-ectomy* is the surgical removal.

18.6
Salpingectomy is the removal of the ovarian ducts, or tubes.

This word is composed of two parts: *salping-* is from the Greek word for tube; and *-ectomy* refers to surgical removal. These are the tubes that allow the eggs to move from the ovary to the womb.

18.7
Colpopexy is the surgical fixation of the vagina.

Colpopexy is made of two words: *colpo-* refers to the vagina; *-pexy* refers to the surgical fixation of a body part.

When Dr. Sharp uses an instrument to visually examine the vagina the procedure is called a colposcopy.

18.8
Salpingopexy is the surgical fixation of the ovarian tube.

Salpingo- is the ovarian tube. *-pexy* means the surgical fixation of a body part.

18.9
Oophoropexy is fixing the ovary in place in the body.

Oophoropexy is made up of two major word parts: *oophor-* refers to the ovary and *-pexy* refers to the surgical fixation of a body part.

18.10
Hysterosalpingography is the x-ray examination of the womb and the ovary duct.

Hystero- refers to the womb; *salpingo-* refers to the ovary duct; and *-graphy* refers to the x-ray exam.

18.11

For his next patient, Dr. Sharp removes the neck of the uterus, where the uterus connects to the vagina. What is this procedure?

_____ Hysterectomy   _____ Cervicectomy   _____ Trachelorrhaphy

18.12

Dr. Sharp is examining his patient's fallopian tube. What's another name for this body part?

_____ Ovarian duct   _____ Inner lining of uterus   _____ Neck of the uterus

18.13

Which term is another word for cervicectomy, the removal of the neck of the uterus?

_____ Salpingectomy   _____ Hysterectomy   _____ Trachelectomy

18.14

Dr. Sharp must suture the neck of the uterus. It was torn. What is the name of this procedure?

_____ Colporrhaphy   _____ Cervicotomy   _____ Trachelorrhaphy

18.15

Dr. Sharp must remove a fibroid tumor from the uterus. What's this procedure?

_____ Hysterectomy
_____ Myomectomy
_____ Culpectomy

CLUE The clue is fibroid tumor. A fibroid tumor is made of muscle tissue. You learned the term for muscle on page 43!

18.11

Cervicectomy is the operation to remove the neck of the uterus.

Cervicectomy is made up of two major word parts: *cervice-* refers to the neck of any body part, and *-ectomy* refers to the surgical removal of that part.

18.12

Fallopian tube is a common name for the ovarian duct.

18.13

Trachelectomy is another term for the surgical removal of the neck of the uterus.

trachel- refers to neck, and *-ectomy* means the surgical removal of a body part.

Take Note!

Trachel- refers to neck or the neck of an organ. Trachea comes from the same word part.

18.14

Trachelorrhaphy is the operation to suture the neck of the uterus.

trachelo- refers to neck; and, *-rrhaphy* is the surgical suturing of a body part.

18.15

A fibroid tumor is made up of muscle tissue; thus, a myomectomy is the removal of the muscle which has become a fibroid tumor.

myom- refers to muscle, and *-ectomy* means surgical excision.

Here's some more terms you will be adding to your knowledge.

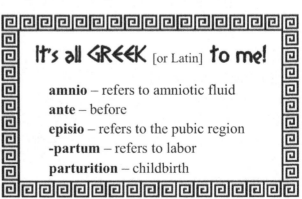

It's all GREEK [or Latin] **to me!**

amnio – refers to amniotic fluid
ante – before
episio – refers to the pubic region
-partum – refers to labor
parturition – childbirth

18.16
What is a medical term for childbirth?

_____ Antepartum   _____ Parturition   _____ Postpartum

18.17
Dr. Sharp provides all the care for his patient during her pregnancy before birth. What's the name of this care?

_____ Antepartum care   _____ Postpartum care   _____ Parturition

18.18
Dr. Sharp's patient is pregnant. Using a needle and syringe, he is removing some fluid from the womb to test for genetic disorders. What's this procedure?

_____ Amniocentesis   _____ Episiotomy   _____ Hysterotomy

18.19
Dr. Sharp provides care for the mother after childbirth. What's this called?

_____ Antepartum care   _____ Postpartum care   _____ Parturition

18.20
Dr. Sharp performs an episiotomy during childbirth. What's this procedure?

_____ Incision of   _____ Removal of   _____ Suturing of
     perineum   perineum   perineum

Quick Review

-tasis = stretching	*-ectasia* = to dilate or stretch
-ptosis = dropping	*-schisis* = separation

18.16

Parturition is the act of giving birth; it is childbirth or the delivery of the baby. It's from the Latin word for labor.

18.17

Antepartum care is medical care prior to giving birth.

Antepartum is made up of two word parts: *ante-* means before; *-partum* means labor. Remember parturition? It means childbirth. It's the same root.

18.18

Amniocentesis is removing fluid from the womb using a needle and syringe.

Amniocentesis is made up of two major word parts: *amnio-* which refers to the amniotic fluid in the womb, and *-centesis* which refers to the use of the needle to extract fluid.

18.19

Postpartum care is the care a doctor provides the mother after birth.

Postpartum is made up of two major word parts: *post-* means after and *-partum* comes from parturition, meaning childbirth.

18.20

An episiotomy is an incision into the perineum tissue, the external area between the vulva and the anus, to keep the baby from tearing the tissue.

Episio- is from the Greek for the pubic region and *–tomy* means incision.

How about a few more terms while we are in this chapter?

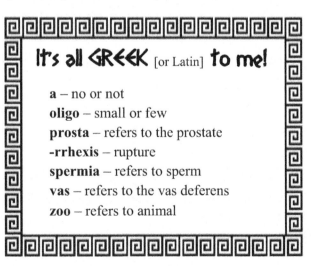

It's all GREEK [or Latin] **to me!**

a – no or not
oligo – small or few
prosta – refers to the prostate
-rrhexis – rupture
spermia – refers to sperm
vas – refers to the vas deferens
zoo – refers to animal

QUICK QUIZ *(Answers in Appendix A)*

_____ 18.9 Oophorectomy   **A.** The surgical removal of the vagina

_____ 18.10 Salpingectomy   **B.** The surgical removal of the ovaries, or of an ovary

_____ 18.11 Colpectomy   **C.** An operation to remove the neck of the uterus

_____ 18.12 Cervicectomy   **D.** The removal of the ovarian ducts, or tubes

18.21

After delivery Dr. Sharp stitches the incision made into the perineum. What's this procedure?

_____ Colporrhaphy   _____ Myomectomy   _____ Episiorrhaphy

18.22

During childbirth, the patient's vagina was torn. What's this called?

_____ Colpostenosis   _____ Colpoptosis   _____ Colporrhexis

18.23

Dr. Sharp's patient has a swollen fallopian tube. It is protruding through a weak spot in the abdominal wall. What's this called?

_____ Salpingolysis   _____ Salpingocele   _____ Salpingolithiasis

18.24

Dr. Sharp needs to create an artificial opening into the ovary to drain an ovarian cyst. What is this procedure called?

_____ Oophorotomy   _____ Salpingostomy   _____ Oophorostomy

18.25

You've got this! Let's see how much word power you've developed. What is the meaning of salpingostomy?

_____

18.21

Episiorrhaphy is the suturing or stitching of the perineum tissue.

Episio- is from the Greek for the pubic region and *–rrhaphy* means suturing.

18.22

Colporrhexis describes a condition where the walls of the vagina are lacerated, ruptured, or torn.

Colporrhexis is made up of two major word parts: *colpo-* refers to the vagina; and *-rrhexis* means rupture.

18.23

Salpingocele is a swelling in the fallopion tube.

Salpingocele is made up of two word parts: *salpingo-* refers to the ovarian ducts, and *-cele* means swelling.

18.24

Oophorostomy is the creation of an artificial opening into the ovary – in this case to drain an ovarian cyst.

Oophorostomy is made of two word parts: *oophoro–* refers to the ovary and *–stomy* means creating an artificial opening.

18.25

Salpingostomy is creating an artifical opening into a fallopian tube.

Salpingostomy is made of two word parts: *salpingo–* refers to the fallopian tube and *–stomy* means creating an artificial opening.

QUICK QUIZ *(Answers in Appendix A)*

_____ 18.13 Oophoropexy	**A.** The surgical fixation of the vagina
_____ 18.14 Colpopexy	**B.** The surgical fixation of the ovarian tube
_____ 18.15 Hysteropexy	**C.** The surgical fixation of the womb
_____ 18.16 Salpingopexy	**D.** The surgical fixation of the ovary

18.26
Roger has an inflammation of the testicles. What is this condition called?

_____ Orchitis   _____ Prostatotomy   _____ Azoospermia

18.27
Leroy and his wife have not been able to conceive a baby. After some lab work it was determined that Leroy has an absence of viable sperm. What is the correct term for this condition?

_____ Orchitis   _____ Prostatotomy   _____ Azoospermia

18.28
Melvin has six children and has decided he doesn't want anymore. Which of the following is done as a way to produce sterility in males.

_____ Vasectomy   _____ Oligospermia   _____ Prostatectomy

18.29
Dr. Sharp determined that he needs to remove the patient's prostate. What's the name of this procedure?

_____ Vasectomy   _____ Oligospermia   _____ Prostatectomy

18.30
Another patient and his wife have been unable to conceive a baby. The lab work shows that his sperm count is low. What is this condition called?

_____ Vasectomy   _____ Oligospermia   _____ Prostatectomy

18.31
You've got this! Let's see how much word power you've developed. Here's a medical term we haven't shown you yet, but you'll be able to decipher its meaning. What is the meaning of prostatotomy?

_____

18.26

Orchitis is inflammation of the testicles.

Orch- is the medical term for testicle and *–itis* means inflammation.

18.27

The correct term for an absence of viable sperm is azoospermia.

The prefix *a-* means no or not, the term *zoo-* refers to animal and the suffix *-spermia* refers to sperm.

18.28

A vasectomy is done to produce sterility in males.

Vas– refers to the vas deferens and *–ectomy* means to remove.

18.29

Excision of the prostate is prostatectomy.

Prosta- is the prefix indicating the prostate and *–ectomy* indicates an excision. Once again, a t is placed in the middle to make it easier to pronounce.

18.30

The condition of having a low sperm count is oligospermia.

The prefix *oligo-* means small or few and the suffix *-spermia* refers to sperm.

18.31

An incision into the prostate gland is a prostatotomy.

Prosta- indicates the prostate. *–otomy* is the suffix for incision. The extra t in the middle is sometimes added to words make them easier to pronounce.

QUICK QUIZ *(Answers in Appendix A)*

_____ 18.17 Larynx	**A.** Tube from the larynx to the bronchial tube
_____ 18.18 Trachea	**B.** Tube from the back of the nose to the esophagus
_____ 18.19 Pharynx	**C.** Voice box
_____ 18.20 Bronchi	**D.** The two branches of the trachea

Chapter Quiz 1 (Answers in Appendix A)

Choose the correct match.

_____ 18.1 Visual exam of uterus	A. Orchitis
_____ 18.2 Visual exam of vagina	B. Oligospermia
_____ 18.3 An absence of viable sperm	C. Hysteroscopy
_____ 18.4 Suturing the neck of the uterus	D. Azoospermia
_____ 18.5 Having a low sperm count	E. Colpopexy
_____ 18.6 Incision into perineum	F. Colposcopy
_____ 18.7 Rupture of vaginal wall	G. Colporrhexis
_____ 18.8 Fixation of vagina to abdominal wall	H. Trachelorrhaphy
_____ 18.9 Inflammation of the testes	I. Episiotomy
_____ 18.10 Surgical opening of a fallopian tube	J. Salpingostomy

You've got this! Use your new knowledge to decipher these words.

_____ 18.11 Oophoropathy	A. Surgical repair of the ovary
_____ 18.12 Oophoroplasty	B. Suture of the ovary
_____ 18.13 Oophorrhagia	C. Surgical connection of the ureter and the fallopian tube
_____ 18.14 Oophorrhaphy	D. Surgical repair of the vagina and perineum
_____ 18.15 Colpostenosis	E. Narrowing of the vagina
_____ 18.16 Salpingosalpingostomy	F. Hemorrhage from the ovary
_____ 18.17 Colpoperineoplasty	G. Any disease of the ovary
_____ 18.18 Salpingo-ureterostomy	H. The operation of attaching one fallopian tube to the other

Write-in the correct word from the list below.

18.19 Excision of the prostate gland _____

18.20 An incision into the prostate gland _____

18.21 Taking an x-ray of ovarian duct and womb _____

18.22 Removal of fibroid tumor _____

18.23 Surgical removal of the womb _____

18.24 The surgical removal of the vagina _____

18.25 Fallopian tube _____

18.26 Childbirth _____

18.27 After childbirth _____

18.28 Creation of an artificial opening into the ovary _____

Myomectomy	Postpartum	Hysterectomy
Oophorostomy	Parturition	Prostatotomy
Prostatectomy	Ovarian duct	Colpectomy
Hysterosalpingography		

Chapter Quiz 2 (Answers in Appendix A)

Choose the correct match.

_____ 18.29 Ovarian duct	A. Creation of an artificial opening into the ovary
_____ 18.30 Postpartum	B. Fallopian tube
_____ 18.31 Prostatotomy	C. The surgical removal of the vagina
_____ 18.32 Myomectomy	D. After childbirth
_____ 18.33 Hysterosalpingography	E. X-ray of womb and ovarian duct
_____ 18.34 Hysterectomy	F. Childbirth
_____ 18.35 Parturition	G. Incision into the prostate gland
_____ 18.36 Colpectomy	H. Removal of fibroid tumor
_____ 18.37 Prostatectomy	I. Surgical removal of the womb
_____ 18.38 Oophorostomy	J. Excision of the prostate gland

You've got this! Use your new knowledge to decipher these words.

_____ 18.39 Oophoralgia	A. Vaginal pain
_____ 18.40 Colpalgia	B. Surgical repair of the neck of the uterus
_____ 18.41 Oophorosalpingitis	C. Pain in an ovary
_____ 18.42 Colpocystitis	D. Suture of the fallopian tube
_____ 18.43 Trachelopexy	E. Inflammation of the ovary and oviduct
_____ 18.44 Tracheloplasty	F. Surgical repair of the fallopian tube
_____ 18.45 Salpingoplasty	G. Surgical fixation of the neck of the uterus
_____ 18.46 Salpingorrhaphy	H. Inflammation of the vagina and bladder

Write-in the correct word from the list below.

18.47 Fixation of vagina to abdominal wall _____

18.48 Having a low sperm count _____

18.49 Surgical opening of a fallopian tube _____

18.50 Visual exam of vagina _____

18.51 An absence of viable sperm _____

18.52 Inflammation of the testes _____

18.53 Rupture of vaginal wall _____

18.54 Incision into perineum _____

18.55 Visual exam of uterus _____

18.56 Suturing the neck of the uterus _____

Colpopexy	Azoospermia	Episiotomy
Colposcopy	Oligospermia	Hysteroscopy
Orchitis	Colporrhexis	Trachelorrhaphy
Salpingostomy		

19

The Nervous System:
Are you nervous?

In the last lesson, you learned some basic words used when describing diseases of and treatment for the reproductive system. In this lesson we'll focus on common terms used with the nervous system.

It's all GREEK [or Latin] to me!

en – inside
mening – refers to the meninges
neur – refers to nerve

19.1
Nerves carry impulses from all parts of the body to the brain and vice versa. What's the term for softening of a nerve?

_____ Meningitis   _____ Neuromalacia   _____ Myelography

19.2
The brain is made up of nerve cells. Sometimes these cells become inflamed. What's this condition?

_____ Otitis   _____ Myelitis   _____ Encephalitis

19.3
The spinal cord is another major part of the nervous system. Sometimes its cells become inflamed. What's this condition?

_____ Otitis   _____ Myelitis   _____ Encephalitis

19.4
The brain is surrounded by connective tissue that protects it. Sometimes these cells become inflamed. What's this condition?

_____ Neuritis   _____ Meningitis   _____ Encephalitis

19.1

<u>Neuromalacia</u> is the term for softening of a nerve.

Neuro- comes from neuron, the Greek word for a nerve and *–malacia* means softening.

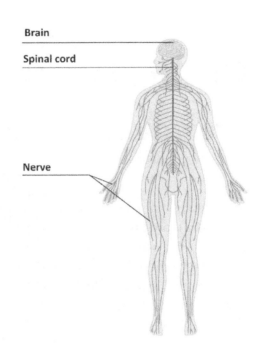

Brain

Spinal cord

Nerve

19.2

<u>Encephalitis</u> is the inflammation of the brain cells.

en- means inside, *cephal-* means head or brain, and *-itis* means inflammation.

19.3

<u>Myelitis</u> is the inflammation of the spinal cord.

Myelitis is composed of two word parts: *myel-* refers to the spinal cord; and *-itis* refers to inflammation. Note: *myel-* also refers to bone marrow. It is used for both body parts.

19.4

<u>Meningitis</u> is the inflammation of the connective tissue that surrounds and protects the brain.

Meningitis is made up of two major word parts: *mening-* refers to the meninges which surround the brain and spinal cord. There are 3 meninges. They are made of connective tissue and they protect the nerves. And, *-itis* = inflammation.

And now for a few more medical terms.

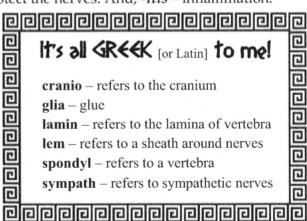

It's all GREEK [or Latin] to me!

cranio – refers to the cranium
glia – glue
lamin – refers to the lamina of vertebra
lem – refers to a sheath around nerves
spondyl – refers to a vertebra
sympath – refers to sympathetic nerves

_____ 19.1 -*rrhexis*   **A.** Suturing

_____ 19.2 –*pexy*   **B.** Rupture

_____ 19.3 -*rhaphy*   **C.** Incision

_____ 19.4 -*tomy*   **D.** Fixation

19.5

Dr. Sharp does a diagnostic test to check his patient's brain waves. What did Dr. Sharp do?

_____ Myelography   _____ Electroencephalography   _____ Cardiography

19.6

Dr. Sharp does a diagnostic test to check his patient's spinal cord. What did Dr. Sharp do?

_____ Myelography   _____ Electroencephalography   _____ Cardiography

19.7

Dr. Sharp's patient has a tumor made of peripheral nerves. What's this condition?

_____ Neurilemoma   _____ Angioma   _____ Lipoma

19.8

Dr. Sharp's patient has a tumor of the brain. What's the name of this condition?

_____ Neurilemoma   _____ Myelocystocele   _____ Encephaloma

19.9

Dr. Sharp's patient has a tumor of the connective tissues of the nerves. What does Dr. Sharp call this condition?

_____ Encephaloma   _____ Glioma   _____ Myelocystocele

19.10

Dr. Sharp's patient has a tumor in the spinal cord. What's this condition?

_____ Encephaloma   _____ Angioma   _____ Myelocystocele

19.5
An <u>electroencephalography</u> shows the brain waves of the patient. A common way of talking about this test is to call it an EEG.

Electroencephalography is made up of 4 word parts: *electro-* refers to electric, *en-* refers to inside, *cephalo-* refers to the head, and *-graphy* refers to an exam that provides a record.

19.6
<u>Myelography</u> is an x-ray to check the spinal cord.

Myelography is made up of two word parts: *myelo-* refers to the spinal cord, and *-graphy* refers to an exam that provides a record.

19.7
A tumor made of peripheral nerves is a <u>neurilemoma</u>.

Neurilemoma is made up of three word parts: *neuri-* refers to the nerve, *lem-* refers to a sheath around the nerve, and *-oma* refers to tumor.

19.8
<u>Encephaloma</u> is a tumor inside the head, or a brain tumor.

Encephaloma is made of three word parts: *en-* refers to inside, *cephal-* refers to the head, *-oma* refers to a tumor.

19.9
A <u>Glioma</u> is a tumor made of neuroglia cells.

Neuroglia cells are the tissue that supports the nervous system, such as cells and fibers. *-glia* means glue.

19.10
<u>Myelocystocele</u> is a cystic tumor of the spinal cord.

Myelocystocele is made of three major word parts: *myelo-* refers to the spinal cord; *cysto-* refers to a bag of fluid, a cyst; and *-cele* refers to a swelling or tumor.

19.11
Dr. Sharp's new patient has a tumor in the meninges. What's this condition?

_____ Encephalopathy   _____ Neuroma   _____ Meningioma

19.12
To operate on the brain, often the doctor must make an incision into the skull. What's this procedure?

_____ Neuroplasty   _____ Craniotomy   _____ Myelotomy

19.13
Dr. Sharp's new patient has problems with her back. He suggests they take out one of the posterior arches of her vertebra. What does Dr. Sharp call this procedure?

_____ Neurectomy   _____ Laminectomy   _____ Myectomy

19.14
Dr. Sharp's new patient has problems with the sympathetic nerves in her neck. Dr. Sharp severs the pathway by cutting out a section of the nerves. What's this procedure called?

_____ Laminectomy   _____ Myectomy   _____ Sympathectomy

19.15
Dr. Sharp's new patient has a defect in the skull. Part of the meninges is protruding through this cavity. What's the name of this condition?

_____ Meningocele   _____ Glioma   _____ Meningomalacia

19.16
Dr. Sharp's patient has a disease that affects his vertebra. It's degenerative arthritis. What's the name of this condition?

_____ Neuralgia
_____ Cephaledema
_____ Spondylosis

CLUE

Check out the prefix for vertebra in the box on page 294!

19.11

A tumor in the meninges is <u>meningioma</u>.

Meningioma is made up of two word parts: *meningi-* refers to the meninges, the three membranes that protect and surround the brain and the spinal cord, and *-oma* refers to a tumor.

19.12

<u>Craniotomy</u> is an incision through the cranium. It is usually done so that the doctor can reach the brain tissue or the meninges tissue.

Craniotomy is made up of two words: *cranio-* refers to the cranium, the part of the skull that encases the brain, and *-tomy* refers to a surgical incision.

19.13

<u>Laminectomy</u> is the removal of the back arch of a vertebra of the spine.

Laminectomy is made up of two word parts: *lamin-* refers to the lamina, a part of the vertebra of the spine, the flat back of the arch of the spine, and *-ectomy* refers to the surgical removal of a body part.

19.14

A <u>sympathectomy</u> involves cutting out part of the nerve path. It is usually done to control pain.

Sympathectomy is made up of two major word parts: *sympath-* refers to the sympathetic nerve system, and *-ectomy* is the surgical excision of a body part.

19.15

<u>Meningocele</u> is part of the meninges pushing through a defect in the skull.

Meningocele is made up of two major word parts: *meningo-* refers to the meninges, the membranes that surround the brain and spinal cord, and *-cele* refers to a swelling.

19.16

<u>Spondylosis</u> is arthritis of the vertebra.

Spondylosis is made up of two major word parts: *spondyl-* is a Greek word for vertebra, and *-osis* means condition.

And, a couple more terms to finish up this chapter.

It's all GREEK [or Latin] to me!

-**dynia** –pain
-**plegia** – stroke or paralysis

19.17
Dr. Sharp's patient is experiencing pain in a vertebra. What's this condition?

_____ Spondylodynia   _____ Cephalgia   _____ Spondylotomy

19.18
The next patient Dr. Sharp sees has a CSF Leak. What's CSF?

_____ Ceruminolytic Agent
_____ Cerebrovascular Accident
_____ Cerebrospinal Fluid

19.19
Dr. Sharp sees a patient whose CSF has accumulated in the brain. What condition does this patient have?

_____ Hydrocephalus   _____ Myelitis   _____ Cephalocele

19.20
Dr. Sharp's next patient's head and neck muscles are paralyzed. What does Dr. Sharp call this condition?

_____ Encephalitis   _____ Cephalodynia   _____ Cephaloplegia

19.21
You've got this! Let's see how much word power you've developed. Here's a medical term we haven't shown you yet, but you'll be able to decipher its meaning. What is the meaning of encephalomyeloneuropathy?

_____

19.17

Spondylodynia is pain in the vertebra.

Spondylodynia is made up of two major word parts: *spondylo-* refers to the vertebra, and *-dynia* refers to pain.

19.18

Cerebrospinal fluid is a water cushion that protects the brain and spinal cord.

Cerebrospinal fluid is commonly referred to as CSF. C stands for cerebro (relating to the brain), S stands for spinal, and F stands for fluid.

19.19

Hydrocephalus is the accumulation of water, or CSF, in the brain.

The CSF is a watery cushion for the brain and spine. *Hydro-* means water and *-cephalus* refers to the brain.

19.20

Cephaloplegia is the paralysis of muscles of the head and/or neck.

Cephaloplegia is made up of two major word parts: *cephalo-* refers to the head, and *-plegia* refers to a stroke or paralysis.

19.21

Encephalomyeloneuropathy is a disease of the brain, spinal cord, and nerves.

Encephalomyeloneuropathy is made up of 4 word parts: *encephalo-* refers to the brain, *myelo-* refers to the spinal cord, *neuro-* refers to the nerves, and *-pathy* refers to any disease.

QUICK QUIZ (Answers in Appendix A)

_____ 19.5 Antrum	**A.** Upon
_____ 19.6 *Epi-*	**B.** To drip
_____ 19.7 Antrotomy	**C.** The cavity in a bone
_____ 19.8 *-staxis*	**D.** The surgical incision into a cavity

---

Chapter Quiz 1 (Answers in Appendix A)

Choose the correct match.

_____ 19.1 Brain tumor	A. Spondylosis
_____ 19.2 Procedure of taking x-ray of the spinal cord	B. Hydrocephalus
_____ 19.3 Protrusion of meninges through a defect in the skull	C. Myelography
_____ 19.4 Arthritis of a vertebra	D. Laminectomy
_____ 19.5 Too much CSF in the brain	E. Meningocele
_____ 19.6 Removal of part of the spinal cord	F. Craniotomy
_____ 19.7 Cutting out part of the nerve path	G. Encephaloma
_____ 19.8 Incision through the cranium	H. Glioma
_____ 19.9 Tumor of the connective tissue of the nerves	I. Sympathectomy

You've got this! Use your new knowledge to decipher these words.

_____ 19.10 Myeloencephalitis	A. Concerning the nervous and renal systems
_____ 19.11 Meningoencephalitis	B. Pain along a nerve
_____ 19.12 Meningomalacia	C. Disease of the brain
_____ 19.13 Myelosclerosis	D. Softening of the meninges
_____ 19.14 Neuroarthropathy	E. Spinal cord and brain inflammation
_____ 19.15 Neuronephric	F. Disease of the joint combined with disease of the nervous system
_____ 19.16 Neuralgia	G. Hardening of the spinal cord
_____ 19.17 Neuromyopathic	H. Pertaining to conditions of the muscles and nerves
_____ 19.18 Encephalopathy	I. Inflammation of the brain and it's meninges

Write-in the correct word from the list below.

19.19 Inflammation of connective tissue
        that surrounds the brain and spinal cord _____

19.20 Paralysis of neck and/or head muscles _____

19.21 Pain in a vertebra _____

19.22 A cystic tumor of the spinal cord _____

19.23 A disease of the brain,
        spinal cord, and nerves _____

19.24 Shows the brain waves of the patient _____

19.25 The basic unit of the nervous system _____

19.26 Inflammation of the brain cells _____

19.27 Inflammation of the spinal cord _____

19.28 A tumor in the meninges _____

Spondylodynia	Myelitis	Electroencephalography
Myelocystocele	Neuron	Encephalomyeloneuropathy
Meningioma	Meningitis	Encephalitis
Cephaloplegia		

Chapter Quiz 2 (Answers in Appendix A)

Choose the correct match.

_____ 19.29 Electroencephalography	A. Inflammation of the spinal cord
_____ 19.30 Meningioma	B. A cystic tumor of the spinal cord
_____ 19.31 Myelitis	C. Inflammation of the brain cells
_____ 19.32 Cephaloplegia	D. Pain in a vertebra
_____ 19.33 Encephalitis	E. A disease of the brain, spinal cord, and nerves
_____ 19.34 Myelocystocele	F. Paralysis of neck and/or head muscles
_____ 19.35 Encephalomyeloneuropathy	G. A tumor in the meninges
_____ 19.36 Meningitis	H. The basic unit of the nervous system
_____ 19.37 Neuron	I. Inflammation of connective tissue that surrounds the brain and spinal cord
_____ 19.38 Spondylodynia	J. Shows the brain waves of the patient

You've got this! Use your new knowledge to decipher these words.

_____ 19.39 Myeloencephalic	A. Any condition of the spinal cord
_____ 19.40 Meningoencephalopathy	B. Concerning the spinal cord and brain
_____ 19.41 Meningoencephalomyelitis	C. Disease of the meninges and brain
_____ 19.42 Myelopathy	D. Inflammation of the brain, spinal cord and their meninges

Write-in the correct word from the list below.

19.43 Incision through the cranium _____

19.44 Cutting out part of the nerve path _____

19.45 Too much CSF in the brain _____

19.46 Arthritis of a vertebra _____

19.47 Disease of the brain _____

19.48 Protrusion of meninges
        through a defect in the skull _____

19.49 Procedure of taking x-ray of the spinal cord _____

19.50 Brain tumor _____

19.51 Tumor of the connective tissue of the nerves _____

19.52 Removal of part of the spinal cord _____

Myelography	Craniotomy	Hydrocephalus
Encephaloma	Encephalopathy	Spondylosis
Glioma	Meningocele	Sympathectomy
Laminectomy		

20

The Musculoskeletal System: Muscles, skeletons and joints (oh, my!)

In this lesson, we'll focus on the musculoskeletal system. Are you ready? Let's go!

It's all GREEK [or Latin] to me!

humer – refers to upper arm bone
olecran – refers to the elbow
phalanges – refers to fingers or toes
scapul – refers to the shoulder blade
uln – refers to the ulna

20.1
What is the medical term for reconstruction of the upper arm?

_____ Claviculectomy   _____ Scapulopexy   _____ Humeroplasty

20.2
Dr. Sharp's next patient has a condition involving his elbow. What's the medical term for any condition involving the elbow joint?

_____ Humeroplasty   _____ Olecranarthropathy   _____ Femurectomy

20.3
The forearm (the lower arm) has two bones. What are their medical terms?

_____ Ulna & radius   _____ Orbit & antrum   _____ Mandible & maxillary

20.4
What is the medical term for the collarbone?

_____ Humerus   _____ Clavicle   _____ Olecranon

20.1

<u>Humeroplasty</u> is reconstruction of the upper arm. Humerus is the Latin word for upper arm. Don't confuse this with humorous, which means funny. They may sound the same, but they have different meanings!

Humero- indicates the humerus and *–plasty* means reconstruction.

20.2

Olecranarthropathy means any condition involving the elbow joint. Olecranon is the Greek word for elbow.

Olecran- indicates the elbow, *arthro-* indicates a joint and *–pathy* means disease.

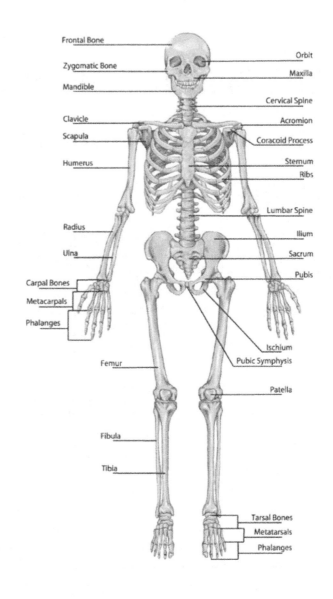

Frontal Bone
Orbit
Zygomatic Bone
Maxilla
Mandible
Cervical Spine
Clavicle
Acromion
Scapula
Coracoid Process
Humerus
Sternum
Ribs
Lumbar Spine
Radius
Ilium
Ulna
Sacrum
Pubis
Carpal Bones
Metacarpals
Phalanges
Ischium
Femur
Pubic Symphysis
Patella
Fibula
Tibia
Tarsal Bones
Metatarsals
Phalanges

Another word for the olecranon is funny bone.
Isn't it interesting that the humerus leads to the funny bone?

20.3

The two bones in the forearm are the <u>ulna & radius.</u>

The ulna is the larger bone; the radius is the smaller bone. It revolves partially around the ulna.

20.4

The <u>clavicle</u> is the collarbone.

Here's a couple more terms.

It's all GREEK [or Latin] to me!

clavicul – refers to the clavicle
teno – refers to tendon

20.5
What's the medical term for pain in the region of the shoulder blade?

_____ Clavicotomy   _____ Humeral   _____ Scapulodynia

20.6
What is the medical term for excision of one or more fingers?

_____ Phalangeal   _____ Phalangectomy   _____ Phalangitis

20.7
Doctor Sharp performs an arthrotomy on his patient to do a biopsy. What did he make an incision into?

_____ Clavicle   _____ Elbow   _____ Ulna

20.8
Dr. Sharp removes part of his patient's collarbone. What did Dr. Sharp do?

_____ A claviculectomy   _____ A scapulopexy   _____ A tenomyotomy

20.9
Dr. Sharp surgically affixes the shoulder blade in place. What did Dr. Sharp do?

_____ A claviculectomy   _____ A scapulopexy   _____ A tenomyotomy

20.10
Dr. Sharp removes part of the tendon in the shoulder area. What did Dr. Sharp do?

_____ A claviculectomy   _____ A capsulorrhaphy   _____ A tenomyotomy

20.11
Dr. Sharp sutures the capsule of the shoulder joint. What does Dr. Sharp call this?

_____ A claviculectomy   _____ A capsulorrhaphy   _____ A tenomyotomy

20.5
Scapulodynia means pain in the region of the shoulder blade.

Scapulo- = refers to the shoulder blade (scapula) and *–dynia* means pain.

20.6
Phalangectomy means excision of one or more phalanges (the fingers or toes). One finger is a phalanx. Another word for phalanges is digit.

Phalang- refers to the phalanges and *–ectomy* means to excise.

20.7
Dr. Sharp made an incision into the patient's elbow.

An arthrotomy is a surgical incision into a joint. The elbow is a joint. The clavicle and the ulna are bones. *Arthr-* refers to joint and *–otomy* means incision.

20.8
Claviculectomy is the surgical removal of the collarbone.

Claviculectomy is made up of two word parts: *clavicul-* refers to the clavicle, or collarbone; and *-ectomy* refers to a surgical removal of a body part.

20.9
Scapulopexy is fixing the shoulder blade in place.

Scapulopexy is made of two word parts: *scapulo-* refers to the shoulder blade, and *-pexy* is the surgical fixation of a body part. In this operation, the doctor attaches the scapula to the ribs.

20.10
A tenomyotomy is the surgical excision of the lateral part of a tendon or muscle.

Teno- refers to tendon, *myo-* refers to muscle, and *-tomy*, in this operation, refers to the incision and removal of a portion of the tendon or muscle.

20.11
Capsulorrhaphy is the surgical suturing of a capsule.

Capsulorrhaphy is made of two word parts: *capsulo-* referring to the capsule that surrounds a joint, and *-rrhaphy* which means to suture.

Let's add these terms to your vocabulary.

It's all GREEK [or Latin] to me!

fascio – membrane around muscles
femor – refers to thigh bone
fibul – refers to small bone in calf
patell – refers to kneecap
tibi – refers to larger bone in calf

20.12

Juan has a hernia, or swelling, of the thigh bone. What is this condition?

_____ Femorocele   _____ Patellectomy   _____ Osteoplasty

20.13

Dr. Sharp had to perform a surgical reconstruction of the patient's kneecap. What does Dr. Sharp call this procedure?

_____ Femorocele   _____ Patelloplasty   _____ Arthrotomy

20.14

Lydia has pain in the shin bone. What does Dr. Sharp call this?

_____ Tibialgia   _____ Femorocele   _____ Phalangitis

20.15

Dr. Sharp surgically removed the knee cap. What did he do?

_____ Osteoplasty   _____ Arthrotomy   _____ Patellectomy

20.16

Dr. Sharp shortens the femur bone for a patient. What did he do?

_____ Arthrotomy   _____ Patelloplasty   _____ Osteoplasty

20.17

Dr. Sharp makes a surgical incision into the connective tissue, the fibrous membrane that supports the muscles of the thigh. What did he do?

_____ Arthrotomy   _____ Fasciotomy   _____ Osteotomy

20.12
Femorocele is a hernia, or swelling, of
the thigh bone (femur).

Femor- refers to the thigh bone and
–cele means hernia or swelling.

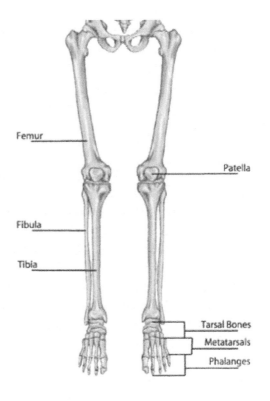

Femur

Patella

20.13
Patelloplasty is reconstruction of the
kneecap (patella).

Patell- refers to the kneecap and
–plasty means reconstruction.

Fibula

Tibia

20.14
Tibialgia is pain in the shin bone.

The tibia is the shin bone, the larger
bone in the calf of the leg. The fibula is
the smaller bone in the calf. *Tibi-*
refers to the tibia and *–algia* means pain.

Tarsal Bones
Metatarsals
Phalanges

20.15
The surgical removal of the kneecap is a patellectomy.

Patellectomy is made up of two words: *patell-* refers to the kneecap, the patella;
and *-ectomy* refers to the surgical removal of a body part.

20.16
Osteoplasty is reforming or reconstructing a bone.

In this case, the doctor reconstructed the bone, by shortening it. Osteoplasty has
two word parts: *osteo-* means bone; *-plasty* means reconstruction or reforming of
a body part. In this scenario, the doctor reformed the femur.

20.17
A surgical incision into the connective tissue is called fasciotomy.

Fasciotomy is made up of two word parts: *fascio-* refers to the fibrous membrane
covering, supporting, and separating muscles, and *-tomy* refers to a surgical
incision.

Just a few more terms before we finish this chapter.

It's all GREEK [or Latin] to me!

tarsal – refers to bones in the foot
tendo – refers to tendon
synov – refers to synovial membrane

20.18

The next patient has a problem with the knee joint. Dr. Sharp surgically removes the membrane that lubricates the joint with fluid. What did he do?

_____ Acetabuloplasty   _____ Arthrocentesis   _____ Synovectomy

20.19

Dr. Sharp's patient has problems with his tibia. Dr. Sharp finds that a fragment of the bone has died. He removes this fragment. What did he do?

_____ Sequestrectomy   _____ Osteoplasty   _____ Arthrotomy

20.20

Dr. Sharp's patient has a fracture. Dr. Sharp makes a surgical incision to the fracture, connects the fractured bone ends and pins them together. What did he do?

_____ Open treatment   _____ Closed treatment   _____ Ostectomy

20.21

Dr. Sharp's patient has adhesions on a tendon. This condition is very painful. It restricts his movement. Dr. Sharp frees the tendons from the adhesions. What did he do?

_____ Tendoplasty   _____ Tendotomy   _____ Tendolysis

20.22

You've got this! Let's see how much word power you've developed. What is the meaning of tarsalgia?

_____

20.18
Synovectomy is removing the membrane that lubricates the joint with fluid.

Synovectomy is made of two major word parts: *synov-* refers to the synovial membrane, the membrane that lines the capsule of a joint and secretes synovia, the lubricating fluid of the joint; and *-ectomy* refers to the surgical removal of a body part.

20.19
Sequestrectomy is when the doctor removes a piece of bone that has died.

Sequestrectomy is made up of two major word parts: *sequestr-* refers to a piece of bone that has died and separated from the live bone, and *-ectomy* refers to the surgical removal of a body part. In this case, Dr. Sharp is removing a piece of the tibia that has died. *Sequestr -* is the Latin word for separate.

20.20
When a doctor repairs a fracture, if s/he makes an incision to open the tissue to the fracture so s/he can see the break and repair it, it is referred to as an open treatment.

When a doctor repairs a fracture without making an incision to the fracture, without visually looking at the fracture, it is referred to as a closed treatment. In this case the doctor may feel the bones and place them without visually looking at the bone.

20.21
Tendolysis is freeing of tendons from adhesions.

Tendolysis is made up of two word parts: *tendo-* refers to a tendon; and *-lysis* refers to the surgical procedure for freeing a body part from adhesions. An adhesion is a fibrous band that sometimes forms and binds a body part.

20.22
Tarsalgia is pain in one of the tarsal bones in the foot.

The tarsal bones are located in the foot. *Tars-* refers to the tarsal bones and *–algia* refers to pain.

The bones in the foot are the tarsals, the metatarsals and the phalanges. Do you remember that the fingers and toes are both called phalanges?

Chapter Quiz 1 (Answers in Appendix A)

Choose the correct match.

_____ 20.1 The collarbone	A. Clavicle
_____ 20.2 Reconstruction of the upper arm bone	B. Femorocele
_____ 20.3 Pain in the larger calf bone	C. Humeroplasty
_____ 20.4 The knee cap	D. Scapulopexy
_____ 20.5 Surgical fixation of the shoulder blade	E. Tibialgia
_____ 20.6 Incision to dissect connective tissue around muscle	F. Phalanges
_____ 20.7 Fingers or toes	G. Capsulorrhaphy
_____ 20.8 Hernia or swelling of the thigh bone	H. Patellectomy
_____ 20.9 Removal of the knee cap	I. Patella
_____ 20.10 The surgical suturing of a capsule	J. Fasciotomy

You've got this! Use your new knowledge to decipher these words.

_____ 20.11 Scapulohumeral	A. Pertaining to the scapula and clavicle
_____ 20.12 Scapuloclavicular	B. Surgical repair of the fascia
_____ 20.13 Scapulalgia	C. Surgical repair of a capsule
_____ 20.14 Capsuloplasty	D. Surgical fixation of the kneecap
_____ 20.15 Tenomyoplasty	E. Inflammation of a synovial membrane
_____ 20.16 Synovitis	F. Pain in the region of the shoulder blade
_____ 20.17 Patellapexy	G. Repair of a tendon and muscle
_____ 20.18 Fasciaplasty	H. Concerning the scapula and humerus

Write-in the correct word from the list below.

20.19 Removal of dead fragment of bone _____

20.20 Removal of membranes that lubricate a joint _____

20.21 Manual manipulation to align a fractured bone _____

20.22 Excision of a finger _____

20.23 The elbow _____

20.24 Freeing of tendons from adhesions _____

20.25 Removal of all or part of the collar bone _____

20.26 Reconstructing a bone _____

20.27 Incision into a tendon and muscle _____

20.28 Repairing a fracture by making
          an incision to open the tissue _____

Tenomyotomy	Synovectomy	Open treatment
Olecranon	Closed treatment	Osteoplasty
Phalangectomy	Claviculectomy	Sequestrectomy
Tendolysis		

Chapter Quiz 2 (Answers in Appendix A)

Choose the correct match.

_____ 20.29 Tenomyotomy	A. Excision of a finger
_____ 20.30 Open treatment	B. Removal of dead fragment of bone
_____ 20.31 Olecranon	C. Removal of membranes that lubricate a joint
_____ 20.32 Synovectomy	D. Reconstructing a bone
_____ 20.33 Phalangectomy	E. Manual manipulation to align a fractured bone
_____ 20.34 Claviculectomy	F. Removal of all or part of the collar bone
_____ 20.35 Osteoplasty	G. Incision into a tendon and muscle
_____ 20.36 Sequestrectomy	H. Repairing a fracture by making an incision to open the tissue
_____ 20.37 Tendolysis	I. Freeing of tendons from adhesions
_____ 20.38 Closed treatment	J. The elbow

You've got this! Use your new knowledge to decipher these words.

_____ 20.39 Fasciectomy	A. Repair of a tendon
_____ 20.40 Fascioplasty	B. Inflamed condition of a fascia
_____ 20.41 Fasciorrhaphy	C. Inflammation of a tendon
_____ 20.42 Fascitis	D. Surgical repair of the fascia
_____ 20.43 Tenodynia	E. Excision of a portion of a tendon
_____ 20.44 Tenonectomy	F. Suturing of fascia
_____ 20.45 Tendonitis	G. Surgical excision of fascia
_____ 20.46 Tendoplasty	H. Pain in a tendon

Write-in the correct word from the list below.

20.47 The knee cap _____

20.48 Reconstruction of the upper arm bone _____

20.49 Fingers or toes _____

20.50 Incision to dissect
        connective tissue around muscle _____

20.51 Hernia or swelling of the thigh bone _____

20.52 Pain in the larger calf bone _____

20.53 The collarbone _____

20.54 Removal of the knee cap _____

20.55 The surgical suturing of a capsule _____

20.56 Surgical fixation of the shoulder blade _____

Phalanges	Clavicle	Patella
Capsulorrhaphy	Patellectomy	Fasciotomy
Humeroplasty	Femorocele	Tibialgia
Scapulopexy		

Word Tour 4

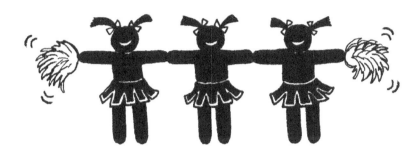

Congratulations! You've made it to the finish. You should be proud of yourself! Take a moment to relax and pat yourself on the back.

Then, when you're ready, forge ahead to these review exercises. Working through these exercises will help you remember the things you've learned.

The questions are organized into two parts. You can work them one page at a time and check your answers with each page, or challenge yourself and check your answers after each part.

So, take a moment, then grab your pencil and get started!

NOTES...

Word Tour 4

Part 1 (Answers in Appendix A)

Match the definitions to the terms.

_____ 4.1 Visual examination of the throat	A. Vagotomy
_____ 4.2 Surgical incision through vagus nerve	B. Pharyngogastrostomy
_____ 4.3 Reforms the upper part of stomach around the esophagus	C. Cholangioma
_____ 4.4 Surgical connection of the throat and the stomach	D. Pharyngoscopy
_____ 4.5 Muscle ring between the esophagus and the stomach	E. Cholecystalgia
_____ 4.6 Uppermost part of stomach	F. Dysphagia
_____ 4.7 Operation to repair part of the stomach that opens into duodenum	G. Achalasia
_____ 4.8 Inability to swallow	H. Pyloroplasty
_____ 4.9 Inability of the muscle to relax	I. Fundoplasty
_____ 4.10 Removal of the bottom part of the stomach	J. Cardiac sphincter
_____ 4.11 A tumor of the bile ducts	K. Fundus
_____ 4.12 Pain in the gall bladder	L. Antrectomy

Write-in the meaning of the term.

4.13 *Chole-* = _____   4.15 *Colp-* = _____

4.14 *Oophor-* = _____   4.16 *Salping-* = _____

Match the definitions to the terms.

_____ 4.17 X-ray showing the gall bladder	A. Myomectomy
_____ 4.18 Surgical connection of the common duct and the small intestines	B. Choledochectomy
_____ 4.19 Surgical connection of the gall bladder and the kidneys	C. Salpingography
_____ 4.20 Freeing of intestinal adhesions	D. Cholecystnephrostomy
_____ 4.21 Surgical connection of the liver and the small intestines	E. Colporrhexis
_____ 4.22 The gall bladder and its ducts	F. Choledochoduodenostomy
_____ 4.23 Removal of the common duct of the gall bladder	G. Enterolysis
_____ 4.24 Gall stones in the common duct	H. Choledocholithiasis
_____ 4.25 Visual exam of vagina	I. Cholecystogram
_____ 4.26 Removal of fibroid tumor	J. Biliary tract
_____ 4.27 Taking an x-ray of ovarian duct	K. Hepaticojejunostomy
_____ 4.28 Rupture of vaginal wall	L. Colposcopy

Write-in the meaning of the term.

4.29 *-ectasia* = _____   4.32 *-dynia* = _____

4.30 *-lysis* = _____   4.33 *-rrhexis* = _____

4.31 *-plegia* = _____   4.34 *-partum* = _____

Match the definitions to the terms.

_____ 4.35 Incision into perineum	A. Neuromyelitis
_____ 4.36 Fixation of vagina to abdominal wall	B. Colpopexy
_____ 4.37 Ovarian tumor	C. Oophorohysterectomy
_____ 4.38 Removal of ovary and uterus	D. Trachelocele
_____ 4.39 Removal of ovary and its duct	E. Spondylosis
_____ 4.40 Swelling of the uterus neck	F. Glioma
_____ 4.41 Removal of part of the spinal cord	G. Oophorosalpingectomy
_____ 4.42 Protrusion of meninges through a defect in the skull	H. Oophoroma
_____ 4.43 Inflammation of nerves and spinal cord	I. Encephalopathy
_____ 4.44 Suturing the ends of a nerve	J. Episiotomy
_____ 4.45 Disease of the brain	K. Neurorrhaphy
_____ 4.46 Tumor of the connective tissue of the nerves	L. Laminectomy
_____ 4.47 Arthritis of a vertebra	M. Meningocele

Write-in the meaning of the term.

4.48 *Cervice-* = _____   4.50 *En-* = _____

4.49 *Trachel-* = _____   4.51 *Myel-* = _____

Match the definitions to the terms.

_____ 4.52 Taking an x-ray of the spinal cord	A. Sequestrectomy
_____ 4.53 Pain in a vertebra	B. Synovectomy
_____ 4.54 Removal of part of the skull	C. Femur
_____ 4.55 Removal of capsule of lens	D. Capsulectomy
_____ 4.56 The upper arm bone	E. Patella
_____ 4.57 Removal of dead bone tissue	F. Olecranon
_____ 4.58 The elbow	G. Tibialgia
_____ 4.59 Incision to dissect connective tissue around muscle	H. Humerus
_____ 4.60 Pain in the larger calf bone	I. Tenomyotomy
_____ 4.61 The thigh bone	J. Fasciotomy
_____ 4.62 Incision into a tendon or muscle	K. Myelography
_____ 4.63 Removal of membranes that lubricate a joint	L. Craniectomy
_____ 4.64 The knee cap	M. Spondylodynia

Write-in the meaning of the term.

4.65 *Lem-* = _____   4.68 *Ante-* = _____

4.66 *Cranio-* = _____   4.69 *Amnio-* = _____

4.67 *Spondyl-* = _____   4.70 *A-* = _____

Word Tour 4

Part 2 (Answers in Appendix A)

Match the terms to the definitions.

_____ 4.1 Pharyngoscopy	A. Inability of the muscle to relax
_____ 4.2 Vagotomy	B. Visual examination of the throat
_____ 4.3 Fundoplasty	C. Muscle ring between the esophagus and the stomach
_____ 4.4 Pharyngogastrostomy	D. Pain in the gall bladder
_____ 4.5 Cardiac sphincter	E. Surgical connection of the throat and the stomach
_____ 4.6 Fundus	F. Surgical incision through vagus nerve
_____ 4.7 Pyloroplasty	G. X-ray showing the gall bladder
_____ 4.8 Dysphagia	H. Uppermost part of stomach
_____ 4.9 Achalasia	I. Operation to repair the part of the stomach that opens into the duodenum
_____ 4.10 Antrectomy	J. Inability to swallow
_____ 4.11 Cholecystalgia	K. Reforms the upper part of stomach around the esophagus
_____ 4.12 Cholecystogram	L. Removal of the bottom part of the stomach

Match the terms to the definitions.

_____ 4.13 Choledochoduodenostomy

_____ 4.14 Cholecystnephrostomy

_____ 4.15 Enterolysis

_____ 4.16 Hepaticojejunostomy

_____ 4.17 Biliary tract

_____ 4.18 Choledochectomy

_____ 4.19 Cholangioma

_____ 4.20 Choledocholithiasis

_____ 4.21 Salpingography

_____ 4.22 Colporrhexis

_____ 4.23 Episiotomy

_____ 4.24 Colpopexy

A. Fixation of vagina to abdominal wall

B. Surgical connection of the liver and the small intestines

C. Removal of the common duct of the gall bladder

D. Rupture of vaginal wall

E. Gall stones in the common duct

F. A tumor of the bile ducts

G. Incision into perineum

H. Surgical connection of the common duct and the small intestines

I. The gall bladder and its ducts

J. Freeing of intestinal adhesions

K. Surgical connection of the gall bladder and the kidneys

L. Taking an x-ray of ovarian duct

Write-in the meaning of the term.

4.25 *Olecran-* = _____

4.26 *Scapulo-* = _____

4.27 *Femu-* = _____

4.28 *Clavicul-* = _____

4.29 *Fascio-* = _____

4.30 *Tarsal-* = _____

Match the terms to the definitions.

_____ 4.31 Oophorohysterectomy	A. Disease of the brain
_____ 4.32 Myomectomy	B. Pain in a vertebra
_____ 4.33 Colposcopy	C. Suturing the ends of a nerve
_____ 4.34 Oophoroma	D. Incision to dissect connective tissue around muscle
_____ 4.35 Trachelocele	E. Removal of ovary and its duct
_____ 4.36 Oophorosalpingectomy	F. Removal of part of the skull
_____ 4.37 Neurorrhaphy	G. Swelling of the uterus neck
_____ 4.38 Encephalopathy	H. Tumor of the connective tissue of the nerves
_____ 4.39 Glioma	I. Visual exam of vagina
_____ 4.40 Spondylodynia	J. Removal of part of the spinal cord
_____ 4.41 Craniectomy	K. Removal of fibroid tumor
_____ 4.42 Laminectomy	L. Removal of ovary and uterus
_____ 4.43 Fasciotomy	M. Ovarian tumor

Write-in the meaning of the term.

4.44 *Laparo-* = _____

4.47 *Antrum-* = _____

4.45 *Sigmoido-* = _____

4.48 *Fundo-* = _____

4.46 *Crico-* = _____

4.49 *Pylor-* = _____

Match the terms to the definitions.

_____ 4.50 Neuromyelitis	A. Removal of capsule of lens
_____ 4.51 Spondylosis	B. Incision into a tendon or muscle
_____ 4.52 Myelography	C. The elbow
_____ 4.53 Meningocele	D. The thigh bone
_____ 4.54 Tenomyotomy	E. Inflammation of nerves and spinal cord
_____ 4.55 Sequestrectomy	F. Taking an x-ray of the spinal cord
_____ 4.56 Tibialgia	G. The upper arm bone
_____ 4.57 Capsulectomy	H. Pain in the larger calf bone
_____ 4.58 Olecranon	I. The knee cap
_____ 4.59 Patella	J. Removal of dead bone tissue
_____ 4.60 Femur	K. Removal of membranes that lubricate a joint
_____ 4.61 Synovectomy	L. Arthritis of a vertebra
_____ 4.62 Humerus	M. Protrusion of meninges through a defect **in** the skull

Write-in the meaning of the term.

4.63 *Glia-* = _____   4.65 *Lamin-* = _____

4.64 *Sympath-* = _____   4.66 *Epision-* = _____

Final Test

Congratulations! You've made it to the Final Test!

There are 100 questions organized into two parts. You can work them one page at a time and check your answers with each page or challenge yourself and check your answers after each part.

These exercises will not only test the knowledge you have gained, they will be a good review to help you cement the new knowledge in memory.

NOTES...

Final Test

Part 1 (Answers in Appendix A)

Match the definitions to the terms.

_____ 1. Visual examination of the throat	A. Pyloroplasty
_____ 2. The surgical suturing of the sac surrounding the heart	B. Osteoporosis
_____ 3. Nose bleed	C. Myopericarditis
_____ 4. Hardening of the artery	D. Otosclerosis
_____ 5. An inflamed vein with blood clot	E. Pericardiorrhaphy
_____ 6. Condition of having calculus in the salivary duct	F. Colostomy
_____ 7. Operation to repair the part of the stomach that opens into the duodenum	G. Arteriosclerosis
_____ 8. Surgical opening in the colon to allow materials to pass outside	H. Cholecystalgia
_____ 9. Fragile bones, easily breakable	I. Pharyngoscopy
_____ 10. Hardening of the bones in the ear causing progressive deafness	J. Sialolithiasis
_____ 11. Pain in the gall bladder	K. Epistaxis
_____ 12. Inflammation of the heart muscle and surrounding sac	L. Thrombophlebitis

Match the definitions to the terms.

_____ 13. Reconstruction of a heart valve

A. Valvuloplasty

_____ 14. A condition where the tissue of the larynx softens

B. Enterolysis

_____ 15. Freeing of intestinal adhesions

C. Gingivectomy

_____ 16. Inflammation of the inner lining of the womb or uterus

D. Pneumopericardium

_____ 17. Severe pain

E. Laryngomalacia

_____ 18. Reconstruction of chamber wall in heart

F. Salpingography

_____ 19. Removal of part of the gum tissue

G. Angina

_____ 20. Gall stones in the common duct

H. Pleurodesis

_____ 21. Taking an x-ray of ovarian duct

I. Osteomyelitis

_____ 22. Surgery that binds the two layers of the pleura together

J. Choledocholithiasis

_____ 23. Inflammation of the bone and bone marrow

K. Septoplasty

_____ 24. Air or gas collected in the sac surrounding the heart

L. Endometriosis

Match the definitions to the terms.

_____ 25. Reconstruction of the ear canal	A. Colposcopy
_____ 26. Procedure for taking an x-ray of the flow of blood through the artery	B. Trachelocele
_____ 27. Pertaining to the kidneys and their blood vessels	C. Cystolithotomy
_____ 28. Visual exam of vagina	D. Cystitis
_____ 29. Excision of the border of the lip	E. Meatotomy
_____ 30. Swelling of the uterus neck	F. Lacrimotomy
_____ 31. Inflammation of the joints (most common type)	G. Vermilionectomy
_____ 32. An incision into the passage into the urethra	H. Arteriography
_____ 33. Tumor of the connective tissue of the nerves	I. Osteoarthritis
_____ 34. Inflammation of the bladder	J. Adenitis
_____ 35. Incision into the tear duct	K. Meatoplasty
_____ 36. Inflammation of the gland	L. Glioma
_____ 37. Incision into bladder to remove stones	M. Renovascular

Match the definitions to the terms.

_____ 38. Excision of a dead part of the bone	A. Dysuria
_____ 39. Inflammation of nerves and spinal cord	B. Cardiomegaly
_____ 40. Enlarged heart	C. Arthrocentesis
_____ 41. Incision into a wall of a bone cavity	D. Patella
_____ 42. Pain in the larger calf bone	E. Tibialgia
_____ 43. Device for examining the urethra and the bladder	F. Sequestrectomy
_____ 44. Difficult or painful urination	G. Olecranon
_____ 45. Removal of the fluid from the joint using a hollow needle	H. Ureteroenterostomy
_____ 46. Inflammation of the iris and the cornea	I. Cardiomyopathy
_____ 47. Connecting the ureter and small intestines through a surgically created opening	J. Neuromyelitis
_____ 48. The elbow	K. Cystourethroscope
_____ 49. Disease of the muscle of the heart	L. Keratoiritis
_____ 50. The knee cap	M. Antrotomy

Final Test

Part 2 (Answers in Appendix A)

Match the terms to the definitions.

_____ 51. Otosclerosis	A. Surgical opening in the colon to allow materials to pass outside
_____ 52. Osteoporosis	B. Hardening of the artery
_____ 53. Thrombophlebitis	C. Pain in the gall bladder
_____ 54. Pyloroplasty	D. Hardening of the bones in the ear causing progressive deafness
_____ 55. Pharyngoscopy	E. Nose bleed
_____ 56. Colostomy	F. Inflammation of the heart muscle and surrounding sac
_____ 57. Arteriosclerosis	G. Operation to repair the part of the stomach that opens into the duodenum
_____ 58. Epistaxis	H. Fragile bones, easily breakable
_____ 59. Cholecystalgia	I. The surgical suturing of the sac surrounding the heart
_____ 60. Sialolithiasis	J. An inflamed vein with blood clot
_____ 51. Myopericarditis	K. Condition of having calculus in the salivary duct
_____ 62. Pericardiorrhaphy	L. Visual examination of the throat

Match the terms to the definitions.

_____ 63. Gingivectomy	A. Gall stones in the common duct
_____ 64. Pleurodesis	B. Removal of part of the gum tissue
_____ 65. Valvuloplasty	C. A condition where the tissue of the larynx softens
_____ 66. Septoplasty	D. Inflammation of the bone and bone marrow
_____ 67. Laryngomalacia	E. Inflammation of the inner lining of the womb or uterus
_____ 68. Endometriosis	F. Air or gas collected in the sac surrounding the heart
_____ 69. Salpingography	G. Reconstruction of chamber wall in heart
_____ 70. Choledocholithiasis	H. Freeing of intestinal adhesions
_____ 71. Pneumopericardium	I. Surgery that binds the two layers of the pleura together
_____ 72. Enterolysis	J. Severe pain
_____ 73. Osteomyelitis	K. Reconstruction of a heart valve
_____ 74. Angina	L. Taking an x-ray of ovarian duct

Match the terms to the definitions.

_____ 75. Arteriography	A. Excision of the border of the lip
_____ 76. Cystolithotomy	B. Inflammation of the bladder
_____ 77. Lacrimotomy	C. Swelling of the uterus neck
_____ 78. Glioma	D. Inflammation of the joints (most common type)
_____ 79. Vermilionectomy	E. Incision into bladder to remove stones
_____ 80. Meatoplasty	F. An incision into the passage into the urethra
_____ 81. Trachelocele	G. Pertaining to the kidneys and their blood vessels
_____ 82. Renovascular	H. Tumor of the connective tissue of the nerves
_____ 83. Meatotomy	I. Inflammation of the gland
_____ 84. Osteoarthritis	J. Procedure for taking an x-ray of the flow of blood through the artery
_____ 85. Cystitis	K. Visual exam of vagina
_____ 86. Adenitis	L. Reconstruction of the ear canal
_____ 87. Colposcopy	M. Incision into the tear duct

Match the terms to the definitions.

_____ 88. Cystourethroscope	A. Pain in the larger calf bone
_____ 89. Arthrocentesis	B. Incision into a wall of a bone cavity
_____ 90. Olecranon	C. Excision of a dead part of the bone
_____ 91. Ureteroenterostomy	D. Inflammation of the iris and the cornea
_____ 92. Tibialgia	E. Removal of the fluid from the joint using a hollow needle
_____ 93. Sequestrectomy	F. Inflammation of nerves and spinal cord
_____ 94. Patella	G. Difficult or painful urination
_____ 95. Dysuria	H. Device for examining the urethra and the bladder
_____ 96. Cardiomyopathy	I. Connecting the ureter and small intestines through a surgically created opening
_____ 97. Antrotomy	J. The elbow
_____ 98. Cardiomegaly	K. Disease of the muscle of the heart
_____ 99. Neuromyelitis	L. The knee cap
_____ 100. Keratoiritis	M. Enlarged heart

Appendix A

Answers to the Quick Quizzes, Chapter Quizzes and exercises.

Chapter 1
Quick Quiz

1.1 Heart
1.2 Stomach
1.3 Blood
1.4 Anus
1.5 Artery
1.6 Skin

Chapter 1
Chapter Quiz

1.1 A.
1.2 F.
1.3 E.
1.4 B.
1.5 D.
1.6 C.
1.7 G.
1.8 F.
1.9 B.
1.10 G.
1.11 A.
1.12 C.
1.13 D.
1.14 E.
1.15 the procedure of making a recording
1.16 suturing
1.17 inflammation
1.18 instrument used to record
1.19 abnormal flow
1.20 a recording
1.21 Arteriorrhaphy
1.22 Carditis
1.23 Arteritis
1.24 Gastrorrhagia
1.25 Hemorrhage
1.26 Cardiogram
1.27 Cardiograph
1.28 Proctitis
1.29 Arteriography
1.30 Gastritis
1.31 Arteriogram
1.32 Cardiography
1.33 Dermatitis
1.34 Gastrorrhaphy

Chapter 2
Quick Quiz

2.1 Stomach
2.2 Blood
2.3 Anus
2.4 Artery
2.5 Lungs
2.6 Liver
2.7 Kidneys
2.8 Skin

Chapter 2
Chapter Quiz

2.1 K.
2.2 A.
2.3 H.
2.4 J.
2.5 C.
2.6 B.
2.7 G.
2.8 D.
2.9 F.
2.10 I.
2.11 E.
2.12 lungs
2.13 liver
2.14 bone
2.15 joint
2.16 kidney
2.17 windpipe
2.18 B.
2.19 D.
2.20 A.
2.21 C.
2.22 Gastrectomy
2.23 Nephrectomy
2.24 Osteitis
2.25 Hepatotomy
2.26 Hepatectomy
2.27 Nephrorrhaphy
2.28 Arthritis
2.29 Arthrography
2.30 Pneumonia
2.31 Nephritis
2.32 Dermatosis
2.33 Arthrotomy
2.34 Bronchography
2.35 Bronchorrhagia
2.36 Nephrotomy

Chapter 3
Quick Quiz

3.1 Bone
3.2 Windpipe
3.3 Joint
3.4 Liver
3.5 Surgical removal
3.6 Surgical incision

Chapter 3
Chapter Quiz 1

3.1 B.
3.2 F.
3.3 D.
3.4 I.
3.5 G.
3.6 H.
3.7 A.
3.8 C.
3.9 E.
3.10 C.
3.11 B.
3.12 A.
3.13 D.
3.14 G.
3.15 F.
3.16 E.
3.17 I.
3.18 H.
3.19 Angiosclerosis
3.20 Adenopathy
3.21 Angioma
3.22 Hepatocarcinoma
3.23 Angioplasty
3.24 Adenocarcinoma
3.25 Adenectomy
3.26 Osteoma
3.27 Gastrocarcinoma
3.28 Angina

Chapter 3
Chapter Quiz 2

3.29 H.
3.30 I.
3.31 G.
3.32 C.
3.33 A.
3.34 J.
3.35 F.
3.36 D.
3.37 B.
3.38 E.
3.39 F.
3.40 G.
3.41 E.
3.42 A.
3.43 B.
3.44 H.
3.45 C.
3.46 D.
3.47 Adenosclerosis
3.48 Blepharitis
3.49 Blepharospasm
3.50 Blepharotomy
3.51 Angiitis
3.52 Blepharoplasty
3.53 Bronchoplasty
3.54 Adenitis
3.55 Bronchospasm
3.56 Blepharorrhaphy

Chapter 4
Quick Quiz

4.1 Head
4.2 Pain or disease
4.3 Ear
4.4 An instrument used for observing or detecting
4.5 Examine using an instrument – a scope
4.6 Refers to the colon
4.7 A surgical opening
4.8 Refers to blood

Chapter 4
Chapter Quiz 1

4.1 C.
4.2 D.
4.3 E.
4.4 B.
4.5 I.
4.6 A.
4.7 G.
4.8 H.
4.9 F.
4.10 J.
4.11 D.
4.12 C.
4.13 H.
4.14 A.
4.15 B.
4.16 J.
4.17 G.
4.18 E.
4.19 I.
4.20 F.
4.21 Hysteroscopy
4.22 Colostomy
4.23 Otoscope
4.24 Proctosigmoido-scopy
4.25 Otoscopy
4.26 Hysterectomy

4.27 Gastrostomy
4.28 Hysterotomy
4.29 Otoplasty
4.30 Cephalhematoma

Chapter 4
Chapter Quiz 2

4.31 I.
4.32 D.
4.33 J.
4.34 B.
4.35 C.
4.36 G.
4.37 F.
4.38 A.
4.39 E.
4.40 H.
4.41 D.
4.42 F.
4.43 E.
4.44 A.
4.45 C.
4.46 H.
4.47 G.
4.48 B.
4.49 Colitis
4.50 Otalgia
4.51 Bronchoscopy
4.52 Otitis
4.53 Cardiomegaly
4.54 Arthroscopy
4.55 Cephalalgia
4.56 Cardiomyopathy
4.57 Gastroscopy
4.58 Arthralgia

Chapter 5
Quick Quiz

5.1 Ear
5.2 Muscle
5.3 Uterus or Womb
5.4 Head
5.5 Gland

5.6 Blood and lymph vessels
5.7 Joint
5.8 Eyelid

Chapter 5
Chapter Quiz 1

5.1 G.
5.2 I.
5.3 F.
5.4 D.
5.5 H.
5.6 A.
5.7 B.
5.8 J.
5.9 C.
5.10 E.
5.11 C.
5.12 D.
5.13 A.
5.14 F.
5.15 J.
5.16 B.
5.17 E.
5.18 G.
5.19 I.
5.20 H.
5.21 Dysmenorrhea
5.22 Arthrocentesis
5.23 Osteoporosis
5.24 Mammoplasty
5.25 Endometriosis
5.26 Osteomyelitis
5.27 Phlebotomy
5.28 Uropathy
5.29 Nephrolithiasis
5.30 Gastroduodenitis

Chapter 5
Chapter Quiz 2

5.31 A.
5.32 I.
5.33 E.
5.34 J.
5.35 D.

5.36 C.
5.37 H.
5.38 F.
5.39 G.
5.40 B.
5.41 C.
5.42 A.
5.43 G.
5.44 F.
5.45 B.
5.46 H.
5.47 D.
5.48 E.
5.49 Lipectomy
5.50 Rhinoplasty
5.51 Phlebitis
5.52 Mammogram
5.53 Dyspepsia
5.54 Mammotomy
5.55 Lipoma
5.56 Pericardium
5.57 Hemodialysis
5.58 Rhinitis

Word Tour I –
Part 1

1.1 A.
1.2 J.
1.3 K.
1.4 B.
1.5 C.
1.6 E.
1.7 I.
1.8 H.
1.9 G.
1.10 L.
1.11 F.
1.12 D.
1.13 skin
1.14 anus
1.15 artery
1.16 heart
1.17 lungs

1.18 liver
1.19 H.
1.20 C.
1.21 D.
1.22 B.
1.23 E.
1.24 G.
1.25 J.
1.26 I.
1.27 A.
1.28 K.
1.29 F.
1.30 L.
1.31 joint
1.32 windpipe
1.33 kidney
1.34 blood
1.35 gland
1.36 blood and lymph vessels
1.37 F.
1.38 M.
1.39 B.
1.40 C.
1.41 L.
1.42 A.
1.43 D.
1.44 H.
1.45 I.
1.46 E.
1.47 J.
1.48 G.
1.49 K.
1.50 abnormal flow
1.51 recording of something
1.52 disease
1.53 excision
1.54 hard
1.55 incision
1.56 D.
1.57 E.
1.58 A.

1.59 J.
1.60 G.
1.61 K.
1.62 M.
1.63 L.
1.64 H.
1.65 B.
1.66 F.
1.67 C.
1.68 I.
1.69 disease
1.70 tumor
1.71 reconstruction
1.72 instrument used for observing
1.73 surgical opening
1.74 large

Word Tour I – Part 2

1.1 L.
1.2 A.
1.3 F.
1.4 J.
1.5 D.
1.6 H.
1.7 I.
1.8 K.
1.9 G.
1.10 C.
1.11 B.
1.12 E.
1.13 nose
1.14 small intestines
1.15 bone marrow
1.16 vein
1.17 C.
1.18 E.
1.19 L.
1.20 I.
1.21 B.
1.22 K.
1.23 J.
1.24 G.

1.25 D.
1.26 A.
1.27 H.
1.28 F
1.29 head
1.30 muscle
1.31 diseased
1.32 stone
1.33 fat tissue
1.34 womb
1.35 K.
1.36 L.
1.37 J.
1.38 H.
1.39 M.
1.40 G.
1.41 F.
1.42 A.
1.43 D.
1.44 B.
1.45 I.
1.46 E.
1.47 C.
1.48 digestion
1.49 disease
1.50 puncture with a hollow needle
1.51 examining using a scope
1.52 pain
1.53 speech (reading)
1.54 L.
1.55 J.
1.56 E.
1.57 I.
1.58 A.
1.59 D.
1.60 K.
1.61 C.
1.62 G.
1.63 M.
1.64 F.
1.65 H.

1.66 B.

Chapter 6
Quick Quiz

6.1 D.
6.2 C.
6.3 B.
6.4 A.
6.5 C.
6.6 A.
6.7 D.
6.8 B.
6.9 D.
6.10 C.
6.11 B.
6.12 A.

Chapter 6
Chapter Quiz 1

6.1 A.
6.2 E.
6.3 G.
6.4 C.
6.5 I.
6.6 B.
6.7 F.
6.8 J.
6.9 H.
6.10 D.
6.11 A.
6.12 E.
6.13 D.
6.14 B.
6.15 F.
6.16 G.
6.17 H.
6.18 C.
6.19 Cystolithotomy
6.20 Urethrotrigonitis
6.21 Cystectomy
6.22 Uremia
6.23 Hydronephrosis
6.24 Hydroureter

6.25 Proteinuria
6.26 Ureter
6.27 Urethra
6.28 Cystotomy

Chapter 6
Chapter Quiz 2

6.29 H.
6.30 C.
6.31 F.
6.32 A.
6.33 D.
6.34 B.
6.35 E.
6.36 J.
6.37 I.
6.38 G.
6.39 G.
6.40 E.
6.41 H.
6.42 F.
6.43 B.
6.44 C.
6.45 D.
6.46 A.
6.47 Litholapaxy
6.48 Hydroureter
6.49 Proteinuria
6.50 Ureter
6.51 Ureterocele
6.52 Cystotomy
6.53 Anastomosis
6.54 Urethropexy
6.55 Urethra
6.56 Fulguration

Chapter 7
Quick Quiz

7.1 B.
7.2 D.
7.3 C.
7.4 A.
7.5 C.

7.6 D.
7.7 A.
7.8 B.

Chapter 7
Chapter Quiz 1

7.1 E.
7.2 F.
7.3 I.
7.4 J.
7.5 B.
7.6 A.
7.7 H.
7.8 D.
7.9 C.
7.10 G.
7.11 C.
7.12 B.
7.13 E.
7.14 H.
7.15 G.
7.16 A.
7.17 F.
7.18 D.
7.19 Nephrocutaneous
7.20 Transurethral
7.21 Nephrogenic
7.22 Renal sclerosis
7.23 Urethral
      diverticulum
7.24. Meatotomy
7.25 Vesicourethropexy
7.26 Vesicostomy
7.27 Ureteropyelo-
      graphy
7.28 Vesicocutaneous

Chapter 7
Chapter Quiz 2

7.29 F.
7.30 H.
7.31 J.
7.32 I.
7.33 A.
7.34 B.

7.35 D.
7.36 C.
7.37 E.
7.38 G.
7.39 A.
7.40 E.
7.41 G.
7.42 H.
7.43 D.
7.44 B.
7.45 F.
7.46 C.
7.47 Cystometrogram
7.48 Cystography
7.49 Uretero-
      pyelostomy
7.50 Pyelostomy
7.51 Pyelotomy
7.52 Pyeloureteritis
      cystica
7.53 Vesicouterine
      fistula
7.54 Resection
7.55 Diverticulitis
7.56 Pyelocutaneous

Chapter 8
Quick Quiz

8.1 D.
8.2 B.
8.3 C.
8.4 A.
8.5 C.
8.6 D.
8.7 A.
8.8 B.

Chapter 8
Chapter Quiz 1

8.1 H.
8.2 B.
8.3 F.
8.4 G.

8.5 J.
8.6 A.
8.7 I.
8.8 D.
8.9 C.
8.10 E.
8.11 E.
8.12 H.
8.13 G.
8.14 F.
8.15 C.
8.16 B.
8.17 A.
8.18 D.
8.19 Mitral
      insufficiency
8.20 Valvuloplasty
8.21 Tachycardia
8.22 Mitral Stenosis
8.23 Septostomy
8.24 Valvotomy
8.25 Cardiopulmonary
      bypass
8.26 Pericarditis
8.27 Cardiovascular
8.28 Pericardium

Chapter 8
Chapter Quiz 2

8.29 J.
8.30 F.
8.31 C.
8.32 H.
8.33 G.
8.34 E.
8.35 D.
8.36 B.
8.37 I.
8.38 A.
8.39 F.
8.40 A.
8.41 H.
8.42 B.
8.43 C.

8.44 G.

8.45 E.

8.46 D.

8.47 Defibrillator

8.48 Aortosclerosis

8.49 Pericardiectomy

8.50 Pneumo-
pericardium

8.51 Anomaly

8.52 Vascular

8.53 Myopericarditis

8.54 Carditis

8.55 Thoracotomy

8.56 Bradycardia

Chapter 9
Quick Quiz

9.1 D.

9.2 A.

9.3 B.

9.4 C.

9.5 C.

9.6 D.

9.7 A.

9.8 B.

9.9 A.

9.10 C.

9.11 D.

9.12 B.

9.13 B.

9.14 A.

9.15 D.

9.16 C.

Chapter 9
Chapter Quiz 1

9.1 A.

9.2 C.

9.3 E.

9.4 H.

9.5 D.

9.6 B.

9.7 J.

9.8 G.

9.9 F.

9.10 I.

9.11 C.

9.12 F.

9.13 D.

9.14 E.

9.15 G.

9.16 A.

9.17 H.

9.18 B.

9.19 Renovascular
disease

9.20 Transluminal
atherectomy

9.21 Intrathoracic

9.22 Endarterectomy

9.23 Atherosclerosis

9.24 Ischemia

9.25 Lumen

9.26 Phlebostenosis

9.27 Embolus

9.28 Embolectomy

Chapter 9
Chapter Quiz 2

9.29 A.

9.30 J.

9.31 G.

9.32 D.

9.33 B.

9.34 E.

9.35 I.

9.36 H.

9.37 C.

9.38 F.

9.39 D.

9.40 H.

9.41 A.

9.42 F.

9.43 G.

9.44 C.

9.45 B.

9.46 E.

9.47 Embolism

9.48 Thrombectomy

9.49 Thromboendarter-
ectomy

9.50 Aneurysm

9.51 Thrombo-

9.52 Thrombosis

9.53 Thrombophlebitis

9.54 Angiostenosis

9.55 Aortoplasty

9.56 Aortitis

Chapter 10
Quick Quiz

10.1 D.

10.2 C.

10.3 A.

10.4 B.

10.5 A.

10.6 C.

10.7 B.

10.8 D.

10.9 B.

10.10 D.

10.11 C.

10.12 A.

Chapter 10
Chapter Quiz 1

10.1 C.

10.2 D.

10.3 J.

10.4 G.

10.5 I.

10.6 B.

10.7 H.

10.8 A.

10.9 E.

10.10 F.

10.11 B.

10.12 G.

10.13 H.

10.14 F.

10.15 D.

10.16 C.

10.17 E.

10.18 A.

10.19 Septotomy

10.20 Urethropexy

10.21 Aortopexy

10.22 Nephrolithotomy

10.23 Ureteroentero-
stomy

10.24 Angiostenosis

10.25 Phlebitis

10.26 Pericarditis

10.27 Valvotomy

10.28 Mitral Stenosis

Chapter 10
Chapter Quiz 2

10.29 B.

10.30 H.

10.31 E.

10.32 F.

10.33 A.

10.34 J.

10.35 I.

10.36 G.

10.37 D.

10.38 C.

10.39 F.

10.40 A.

10.41 E.

10.42 H.

10.43 D.

10.44 C.

10.45 B.

10.46 G.

10.47 Valvulitis

10.48 Atherectomy

10.49 Myocarditis

10.50 Trigonitis

10.51 Pericardio-
rrhaphy

10.52 Cystitis

10.53 Nephroureter-
    ectomy
10.54 Embolectomy
10.55 Pneumo-
    pericardium
10.56 Pyelitis

Word Tour II - Part 1

2.1 H.
2.2 F.
2.3 A.
2.4 G.
2.5 C.
2.6 I.
2.7 D.
2.8 B.
2.9 J.
2.10 E.
2.11 L.
2.12 K.
2.13 bladder
2.14 through
2.15 bladder
2.16 chest
2.17 B.
2.18 F.
2.19 J.
2.20 D.
2.21 C.
2.22 G.
2.23 E.
2.24 H.
2.25 K.
2.26 I.
2.27 L.
2.28 A.
2.29 kidney
2.30 fast
2.31 slow
2.32 space within
    artery
2.33 E.

2.34 H.
2.35 I.
2.36 B.
2.37 C.
2.38 F.
2.39 K.
2.40 D.
2.41 J.
2.42 M.
2.43 L.
2.44 A.
2.45 G.
2.46 a person who
    studies a subject
2.47 arising from
2.48 hold or fasten
2.49 swelling
2.50 B.
2.51 C.
2.52 A.
2.53 E.
2.54 J.
2.55 H.
2.56 G.
2.57 D.
2.58 F.
2.59 I.
2.60 M.
2.61 K.
2.62 L.

Word Tour II - Part 2

2.1 L.
2.2 F.
2.3 A.
2.4 H.
2.5 K.
2.6 J.
2.7 B.
2.8 E.
2.9 G.
2.10 I.

2.11 C.
2.12 D.
2.13 A.
2.14 J.
2.15 B.
2.16 I.
2.17 C.
2.18 D.
2.19 F.
2.20 H.
2.21 K.
2.22 L.
2.23 E.
2.24 G.
2.25 pelvis of kidney
2.26 measure
2.27 blood vessels
2.28 inside
2.29 C.
2.30 D.
2.31 L.
2.32 G.
2.33 F.
2.34 H.
2.35 M.
2.36 K
2.37 A.
2.38 B.
2.39 J.
2.40 I.
2.41 E.
2.42 narrowing
2.43 deficiency of blood
    to a body part
2.44 joining two body
    parts
2.45 removing part of
    an organ
2.46 C.
2.47 A.
2.48 L.
2.49 D.
2.50 I.

2.51 J.
2.52 E.
2.53 K.
2.54 B.
2.55 H.
2.56 M.
2.57 G.
2.58 F.

Chapter 11
Quick Quiz

11.1 A.
11.2 D.
11.3 C.
11.4 B.

Chapter 11
Chapter Quiz 1

11.1 B.
11.2 H.
11.3 A.
11.4 F.
11.5 G.
11.6 J.
11.7 E.
11.8 I.
11.9 D.
11.10 C.
11.11 B.
11.12 C.
11.13 G.
11.14 A.
11.15 H.
11.16 E.
11.17 F.
11.18 D.
11.19 Pleurectomy
11.20 Laryngectomy
11.21 Laryngography
11.22 Trachea
11.23 Laryngograph
11.24 Ethmoiditis
11.25 Laryngogram

11.26 Rhinitis
11.27 Bronchi
11.28 Maxillitis

Chapter 11

Chapter Quiz 2

11.29 D.
11.30 H.
11.31 F.
11.32 A.
11.33 I.
11.34 J.
11.35 E.
11.36 C.
11.37 B.
11.38 G.
11.39 F.
11.40 D.
11.41 A.
11.42 H.
11.43 G.
11.44 E.
11.45 C.
11.46 B.
11.47 Transantral
11.48 Pleura
11.49 Epiglottis
11.50 Pharyngocele
11.51 Epistaxis
11.52 Laryngopharyng-
        ectomy
11.53 Nasopharynx
11.54 Antrotomy
11.55 Pneumatocele
11.56 Antrum

Chapter 12

Quick Quiz

12.1 C.
12.2 A.
12.3 D.
12.4 B.

Chapter 12

Chapter Quiz 1

12.1 H.
12.2 C.
12.3 E.
12.4 D.
12.5 I.
12.6 J.
12.7 G.
12.8 F.
12.9 A.
12.10 B.
12.11 E.
12.12 H.
12.13 A.
12.14 G.
12.15 B.
12.16 C.
12.17 D.
12.18 F.
12.19 Pneumothorax
12.20 Laryngoedema
12.21 Intubation
12.22 Supraglottic
12.23 Tracheostomy
12.24 Hypoxia
12.25 Arytenoidectomy
12.26 Thyroidotomy
12.27 Endotracheal
12.28 Cyanosis

Chapter 12

Chapter Quiz 2

12.29 C.
12.30 F.
12.31 G.
12.32 D.
12.33 J.
12.34 A.
12.35 H.
12.36 E.
12.37 B.
12.38 I.
12.39 F.

13.40 A.
12.41 H.
12.42 C.
12.43 B.
12.44 D.
12.45 E.
12.46 G.
12.47 Lobectomy
12.48 Thoracentesis
12.49 Laryngoplasty
12.50 Thoracostomy
12.51 Tracheotomy
12.52 Laryngomalacia
12.53 Laryngotracheo-
        bronchitis
12.54 Tachypnea
12.55 Tracheostenosis
12.56 Pleurodesis

Chapter 13

Quick Quiz

13.1 A.
13.2 C.
13.3 D.
13.4 B.
13.5 C.
13.6 A.
13.7 B.
13.8 D.
13.9 D.
13.10 A.
13.11 B.
13.12 C.

Chapter 13

Chapter Quiz 1

13.1 H.
13.2 B.
13.3 I.
13.4 C.
13.5 F.
13.6 J.
13.7 A.

13.8 E.
13.9 G.
13.10 D.
13.11 G.
13.12 B.
13.13 E.
13.14 A.
13.15 F.
13.16 H.
13.17 D.
13.18 C.
13.19 Labyrinth
13.20 Tympanic
        Membrane
13.21 Meatoplasty
13.22 Transtympanic
13.23 Cholesteatoma
13.24 Tinnitus
13.25 Cochlea
13.26 Mastoidectomy
13.27 Labyrinthitis
13.28 Myringoplasty

Chapter 13

Chapter Quiz 2

13.29 J.
13.30 A.
13.31 H.
13.32 B.
13.33 I.
13.34 C.
13.35 E.
13.36 F.
13.37 D.
13.38 G.
13.39 A.
13.40 G.
13.41 B.
13.42 D.
13.43 C.
13.44 H.
13.45 E.
13.46 F.
13.47 Stapedotomy

13.48 Pinna
13.49 Tympanotomy
13.50 Otoplasty
13.51 Postauricular
13.52 Mastoid antrum
13.53 Otosclerosis
13.54 Otopharynx tube
13.55 Meatus
13.56 Tympanosclerosis

Chapter 14
Quick Quiz

14.1 A.
14.2 C.
14.3 D.
14.4 B.

Chapter 14
Chapter Quiz 1

14.1 D.
14.2 F.
14.3 B.
14.4 E.
14.5 H.
14.6 C.
14.7 A.
14.8 G.
14.9 B.
14.10 C.
14.11 J.
14.12 L.
14.13 K.
14.14 H.
14.15 F.
14.16 E.
14.17 D.
14.18 G.
14.19 A.
14.20 I.
14.21 Vestibuloplasty
14.22 Sublingual
14.23 Uvulopalato-
       pharyngoplasty

14.24 Sialolithiasis
14.25 Sequestrectomy
14.26 Labioglosso-
       laryngeal
14.27 Gingivitis
14.28 Frenulum
14.29 Sialodochoplasty
14.30 Frenotomy

Chapter 14
Chapter Quiz 2

14.31 G.
14.32 J.
14.33 A.
14.34 C.
14.35 H.
14.36 D.
14.37 I.
14.38 E.
14.39 B.
14.40 F.
14.41 F.
14.42 G.
14.43 A.
14.44 E.
14.45 C.
14.46 H.
14.47 B.
14.48 D.
14.49 Cheilitis
14.50 Glossoptosis
14.51 Vermilionectomy
14.52 Cheiloplasty
14.53 Palatoplasty
14.54 Dentoalveolar
14.55 Sialography
14.56 Hemiglossectomy
14.57 Frenoplasty
14.58 Palatoglossal

Chapter 15
Quick Quiz

15.1 C.

15.2 D.
15.3 B.
15.4 A.
15.5 C.
15.6 B.
15.7 A.
15.8 D.
15.9 D.
15.10 A.
15.11 B.
15.12 C.
15.13 B.
15.14 D.
15.15 A.
15.16 C.

Chapter 15
Chapter Quiz 1

15.1 J.
15.2 C.
15.3 F.
15.4 H.
15.5 I.
15.6 B.
15.7 G.
15.8 E.
15.9 D.
15.10 A.
15.11 A.
15.12 G.
15.13 D.
15.14 B.
15.15 C.
15.16 H.
15.17 F.
15.18 E.
15.19 Phacoplanesis
15.20 Choroidopathy
15.21 Iridoptosis
15.22 Canthotomy
15.23 Epikeratophakia
15.24 Scleromalacia
15.25 Iridocapsul-
       ectomy

15.26 Keratohemia
15.27 Orbitonasal
15.28 Choroidocyclitis

Chapter 15
Chapter Quiz 2

15.29 B.
15.30 G.
15.31 I.
15.32 C.
15.33 A.
15.34 E.
15.35 F.
15.36 J.
15.37 D.
15.38 H.
15.39 D.
15.40 E.
15.41 F.
15.42 A.
15.43 G.
15.44 H.
15.45 C.
15.46 B.
15.47 Iridotasis
15.48 Cyclokeratitis
15.49 Blepharoptosis
15.50 Keratomalacia
15.51 Lacrimotomy
15.52 Orbitotomy
15.53 Iridoschisis
15.54 Blepharedema
15.55 Iridocyclo-
       choroiditis
15.56 Phacosclerosis

Word Tour III -
Part 1

3.1 J.
3.2 B.
3.3 I.
3.4 A.
3.5 F.

3.6 G.

3.7 L.

3.8 C.

3.9 E.

3.10 H.

3.11 D.

3.12 K.

3.13 nose

3.14 oral (mouth)

3.15 under or below

3.16 duct

3.17 I.

3.18 G.

3.19 C.

3.20 B.

3.21 F.

3.22 J.

3.23 H.

3.24 E.

3.25 A.

3.26 L.

3.27 D.

3.28 K.

3.29 ear drum

3.30 lips

3.31 tongue

3.32 tympanic
      membrane

3.33 corners of the eye

3.34 salivary glands

3.35 H.

3.36 J.

3.37 C.

3.38 D.

3.39 F.

3.40 I.

3.41 L.

3.42 E.

3.43 B.

3.44 A.

3.45 M.

3.46 G.

3.47 K.

3.48 softening

3.49 swelling

3.50 breath

3.51 binding together

3.52 stretching

3.53 oxygen

3.54 L.

3.55 K.

3.56 M.

3.57 A.

3.58 D.

3.59 J.

3.60 H.

3.61 I.

3.62 C.

3.63 B.

3.64 F.

3.65 E.

3.66 G.

Word Tour III - Part 2

3.1 C.

3.2 A.

3.3 E.

3.4 J.

3.5 I.

3.6 B.

3.7 D.

3.8 G.

3.9 L.

3.10 K.

3.11 F.

3.12 H.

3.13 A.

3.14 J.

3.15 B.

3.16 I.

3.17 L.

3.18 E.

3.19 D.

3.20 G.

3.21 C.

3.22 F.

3.23 H.

3.24 K.

3.25 lens

3.26 cornea

3.27 after or behind

3.28 blue

3.29 above

3.30 thyroid cartilage

3.31 J.

3.32 I.

3.33 B.

3.34 G.

3.35 F.

3.36 E.

3.37 D.

3.38 K.

3.39 A.

3.40 L.

3.41 H.

3.42 M.

3.43 C.

3.44 below

3.45 teeth

3.46 lips

3.47 half

3.48 dropping

3.49 dripping

3.50 L.

3.51 K.

3.52 M.

3.53 D.

3.54 J.

3.55 H.

3.56 A.

3.57 G.

3.58 B.

3.59 I.

3.60 E.

3.61 F.

3.62 C.

**Chapter 16
Quick Quiz**

16.1 C.

16.2 A.

16.3 D.

16.4 B.

16.5 A.

16.6 B.

16.7 C.

16.8 D.

16.9 C.

16.10 A.

16.11 D.

16.12 B.

16.13 A.

16.14 D.

16.15 B.

16.16 C.

**Chapter 16
Chapter Quiz 1**

16.1 B.

16.2 C.

16.3 E.

16.4 I.

16.5 A.

16.6 F.

16.7 J.

16.8 H.

16.9 D.

16.10 G.

16.11 H.

16.12 A.

16.13 G.

16.14 C.

16.15 F.

16.16 E.

16.17 D.

16.18 B.

16.19 Antrectomy

16.20 Fundoplasty

16.21 Cheilitis

16.22 Sialitis

16.23 Glossitis

16.24 Pharyngoscopy

16.25 Oropharynx

16.26 Pharyngitis

16.27 Esophagoscopy

16.28 Nasopharynx

Chapter 16
Chapter Quiz 2

16.29 I.

16.30 B.

16.31 F.

16.32 H.

16.33 G.

16.34 J.

16.35 C.

16.36 E.

16.37 A.

16.38 D.

16.39 D.

16.40 H.

16.41 F.

16.42 A.

16.43 C.

16.44 G.

16.45 B.

16.46 E.

16.47 Fundoplication

16.48 Pharyngo-
gastrostomy

16.49 Pharynx

16.50 Vagotomy

16.51 Dysphagia

16.52 Fundus

16.53 Pyloroplasty

16.54 Esophagus

16.55 Achalasia

16.56 Cardiac Sphincter

Chapter 17
Quick Quiz

17.1 C.

17.2 A.

17.3 D.

17.4 B.

17.5 C.

17.6 A.

17.7 D.

17.8 B.

17.9 C.

17.10 D.

17.11 A.

17.12 B.

17.13 B.

17.14 D.

17.15 A.

17.16 C.

17.17 C.

17.18 A.

17.19 D.

17.20 B.

17.21 B.

17.22 A.

17.23 D.

17.24 C.

17.25 A.

17.26 B.

17.27 D.

17.28 C.

17.29 D.

17.30 B.

17.31 A.

17.32 C.

Chapter 17
Chapter Quiz 1

17.1 E.

17.2 B.

17.3 F.

17.4 G.

17.5 H.

17.6 A.

17.7 I.

17.8 C.

17.9 D.

17.10 C.

17.11 E.

17.12 A.

17.13 B.

17.14 D.

17.15 Cholangiolitis

17.16 Cholecystopexy

17.17 Pancreato-
lithectomy

17.18 Cholecystitis

17.19 Choledochitis

17.20 Cholecysto-
lithiasis

17.21 Choledocho-
rrhaphy

17.22 Pancreatitis

17.23 Enterolysis

17.24 Ileocolitis

Chapter 17
Chapter Quiz 2

17.25 G.

17.26 H.

17.27 F.

17.28 B.

17.29 A.

17.30 J.

17.31 D.

17.32 C.

17.33 E.

17.34 I.

17.35 C.

17.36 E.

17.37 G.

17.38 A.

17.39 H.

17.40 F.

17.41 B.

17.42 D.

17.43 Cholecystogram

17.44 Cholecystentero
stomy

17.45 Choledoch-
ectomy

17.46 Hepaticojejuno-
stomy

17.47 Choledocho-
duodenostomy

17.48 Ileocolitis

17.49 Cholangioma

17.50 Biliary tract

17.51 Pancreato-
duodenostomy

17.52 Cholangio-
pancreatography

Chapter 18
Quick Quiz

18.1 C.

18.2 A.

18.3 D.

18.4 B.

18.5 A.

18.6 C.

18.7 B.

18.8 D.

18.9 B.

18.10 D.

18.11 A.

18.12 C.

18.13 D.

18.14 A.

18.15 C.

18.16 B.

18.17 C.

18.18 A.

18.19 B.

18.20 D.

Chapter 18
Chapter Quiz 1

18.1 C.

18.2 F.

18.3 D.

18.4 H

18.5 B.

18.6 I.

18.7 G.

18.8 E.

18.9 A.

18.10 J.

18.11 G.

18.12 A.

18.13 F.

18.14 B.

18.15 E.

18.16 H.

18.17 D.
18.18 C.
18.19 Prostatectomy
18.20 Prostatotomy
18.21 Hysterosalpingo - graphy
18.22 Myomectomy
18.23 Hysterectomy
18.24 Colpectomy
18.25 Ovarian duct
18.26 Parturition
18.27 Postpartum
18.28 Oophorostomy

Chapter 18
Chapter Quiz 2

18.29 B.
18.30 D.
18.31 G.
18.32 H.
18.33 E.
18.34 I.
18.35 F.
18.36 C.
18.37 J.
18.38 A.
18.39 C.
18.40 A.
18.41 E.
18.42 H.
18.43 G.
18.44 B.
18.45 F.
18.46 D.
18.47 Colpopexy
18.48 Oligospermia
18.49 Salpingostomy
18.50 Colposcopy
18.51 Azoospermia
18.52 Orchitis
18.53 Colporrhexis
18.54 Episiotomy
18.55 Hysteroscopy
18.56 Trachelorrhaphy

Chapter 19
Quick Quiz

19.1 B.
19.2 D.
19.3 A.
19.4 C.
19.5 C.
19.6 A.
19.7 D.
19.8 B.

Chapter 19
Chapter Quiz 1

19.1 G.
19.2 C.
19.3 E.
19.4 A.
19.5 B.
19.6 D.
19.7 I.
19.8 F.
19.9 H.
19.10 E.
19.11 I.
19.12 D.
19.13 G.
19.14 F.
19.15 A.
19.16 B.
19.17 H.
19.18 C.
19.19 Meningitis
19.20 Cephaloplegia
19.21 Spondylodynia
19.22 Myelocystocele
19.23 Encephalomyelo-neuropathy
19.24 Electroencephalo-graphy
19.25 Neuron
19.26 Encephalitis
19.27 Myelitis
19.28 Meningioma

Chapter 19
Chapter Quiz 2

19.29 J.
19.30 G.
19.31 A.
19.32 F.
19.33 C.
19.34 B.
19.35 E.
19.36 I.
19.37 H.
19.38 D.
19.39 B.
19.40 C.
19.41 D.
19.42 A.
19.43 Craniotomy
19.44 Sympathectomy
19.45 Hydrocephalus
19.46 Spondylosis
19.47 Encephalopathy
19.48 Meningocele
19.49 Myelography
19.50 Encephaloma
19.51 Glioma
19.52 Laminectomy

Chapter 20
Chapter Quiz 1

20.1 A.
20.2 C.
20.3 E.
20.4 I.
20.5 D.
20.6 J.
20.7 F.
20.8 B.
20.9 H.
20.10 G.
20.11 H.
20.12 A.
20.13 F.

20.14 C.
20.15 G.
20.16 E.
20.17 D.
20.18 B.
20.19 Sequestrectomy
20.20 Synovectomy
20.21 Closed Treatment
20.22 Phalangectomy
20.23 Olecranon
20.24 Tendolysis
20.25 Claviculectomy
20.26 Osteoplasty
20.27 Tenomyotomy
20.28 Open treatment

Chapter 20
Chapter Quiz 2

20.29 G.
20.30 H.
20.31 J.
20.32 C.
20.33 A.
20.34 F.
20.35 D.
20.36 B.
20.37 I.
20.38 E.
20.39 G.
20.40 D.
20.41 F.
20.42 B.
20.43 H.
20.44 E.
20.45 C.
20.46 A.
20.47 Patella
20.48 Humeroplasty
20.49 Phalanges
20.50 Fasciotomy
20.51 Femorocele
20.52 Tibialgia
20.53 Clavicle
20.54 Patellectomy

20.55 Capsulorrhaphy

20.56 Scapulopexy

Word Tour IV - Part 1

4.1 D.

4.2 A.

4.3 I.

4.4 B.

4.5 J.

4.6 K.

4.7 H.

4.8 F.

4.9 G.

4.10 L.

4.11 C.

4.12 E.

4.13 bile

4.14 ovaries

4.15 vagina

4.16 ovarian ducts

4.17 I.

4.18 F.

4.19 D.

4.20 G.

4.21 K.

4.22 J.

4.23 B.

4.24 H.

4.25 L.

4.26 A.

4.27 C.

4.28 E.

4.29 dilate or stretch

4.30 freeing of adhesions

4.31 stroke

4.32 pain

4.33 rupture

4.34 labor

4.35 J.

4.36 B.

4.37 H.

4.38 C.

4.39 G.

4.40 D.

4.41 L.

4.42 M.

4.43 A.

4.44 K.

4.45 I.

4.46 F.

4.47 E.

4.48 the neck of a body part

4.49 the neck of a body part

4.50 inside

4.51 spinal cord

4.52 K.

4.53 M

4.54 L.

4.55 D.

4.56 H.

4.57 A.

4.58 F.

4.59 J.

4.60 G.

4.61 C.

4.62 I.

4.63 B.

4.64 E.

4.65 a sheath around the nerve

4.66 cranium

4.67 vertebra

4.68 before

4.69 amniotic fluid

4.70 no or not

Word Tour IV - Part 2

4.1 B.

4.2 F.

4.3 K.

4.4 E.

4.5 C.

4.6 H.

4.7 I.

4.8 J.

4.9 A.

4.10 L.

4.11 D.

4.12 G.

4.13 H.

4.14 K.

4.15 J.

4.16 B.

4.17 I.

4.18 C.

4.19 F.

4.20 E.

4.21 L.

4.22 D.

4.23 G.

4.24 A.

4.25 elbow

4.26 shoulder blade

4.27 thigh bone

4.28 collarbone

4.29 fibrous membrane around muscles

4.30 tarsal bones in foot

4.31 L.

4.32 K.

4.33 I.

4.34 M.

4.35 G.

4.36 E.

4.37 C.

4.38 A.

4.39 H.

4.40 B.

4.41 F.

4.42 J.

4.43 D.

4.44 abdomen

4.45 lower part of the descending colon

4.46 cartilage in larynx

4.47 bottom half of stomach

4.48 top part stomach

4.49 pylorus

4.50 E.

4.51 L.

4.52 F.

4.53 M.

4.54 B.

4.55 J.

4.56 H.

4.57 A.

4.58 C.

4.59 I.

4.60 D.

4.61 K.

4.62 G.

4.63 glue

4.64 sympathetic nervous system

4.65 lamina of spine

4.66 pubic region

Final Test Part 1

1. I.

2. E.

3. K.

4. G.

5. L.

6. J.

7. A.

8. F.

9. B.

10. D.

11. H.

12. C.

13. A.

14. E.

15. B.

16. L.

17. G.

18. K.

19. C.

20. J.
21. F.
22. H.
23. I.
24. D.
25. K.
26. H.
27. M.
28. A.
29. G.
30. B.
31. I.
32. E.
33. L.
34. D.
35. F.
36. J.
37. C.
38. F.
39. J.
40. B.
41. M.
42. E.
43. K.
44. A.
45. C.
46. L.
47. H.
48. G.
49. I.
50. D.

Final Test
Part 2

51. D.
52. H.
53. J.
54. G.
55. L.
56. A.
57. B.
58. E.
59. C.
60. K.

61. F.
62. I.
63. B.
64. I.
65. K.
66. G.
67. C.
68. E.
69. L.
70. A.
71. F.
72. H.
73. D.
74. J.
75. J.
76. E.
77. M.
78. H.
79. A.
80. L.
81. C.
82. G.
83. F.
84. D.
85. B.
86. I.
87. K.
88. H.
89. E.
90. J.
91. I.
92. A.
93. C.
94. L.
95. G.
96. K.
97. B.
98. M.
99. F.
100. D.

Appendix B

Index of Word Parts and Words Covered

Roots, Prefixes, Suffixes and Word Parts

a no or not
al pertaining to
adeno gland
algia pain
alveola refers to teeth sockets
amnio refers to amniotic fluid
angi blood and lymph vessels
ante before
antro refers to a cavity in a bone
aort refers to the aorta
ar pertaining to
arterio indicates artery
arthro joint
athero fatty deposit
auricul indicates auricle, outer ear

blepharo eyelid
brady slow
bronchi pleural for branches in lung
broncho windpipe
bronchus refers to a branch in lung

calculus small stone
cantho refers to corners of the eye
capsul refers to capsule of lens
carcino cancerous
cardio heart
-cele swelling
-centesis puncture with a hollow
    needle
cephalo refers to the head
cerebro relating to the brain

cervice refers to neck of a body part
cheil lips
cholang refers to gall bladder ducts
chole bile
clavicul refers to the clavicle
col refers to the large intestines
colo refers to the colon
colono refers to the colon
colp vagina
conjunctiv refers to the conjunctiva of
    the eye
cranio refers to the cranium
crico refers to cartilage in the larynx
-cutaneous pertaining to the skin
cyan dark blue
cyclo refers to the ciliary body
cyst bladder

dento refers to the teeth
derma skin
-desis binding together
doch refers to a duct
duoden refers to small intestines
-dynia pain
dys bad or diseased

-ectasia to dilate or stretch
-ectomy excision, surgical removal
-edema swelling
embol something that blocks
encephalo refers to inside the head
en inside

endo inside or within
entero refers to small intestines
epi upon
episio refers to the pubic region
esophago refers to the esophagus

fascio membrane around muscles
femu refers to femur, thigh bone
fibul refers to small bone in calf
fundo refers to the top part of the
    stomach

gastro stomach
-genic producing, arising from
gingivi refers to gums
glia glue
gloss tongue
glottic refers to the glottis
-gram something written or drawn
-graph instrument used to record
-graphy the procedure of recording

hemi half
hemo blood
hepato liver
humer refers to upper arm bone
hydro water or watery fluid
hypo under, beneath, below
hystero refers to the uterus

-ia indicates disease or condition
-iasis indicates disease
-ic pertaining to
ileo refers to part of small intestine
intra inside
irido refers to the iris
-ism disease, condition of
ische deficiency of blood
-itis inflammation

jejuno refers to the jejunum, part of
    the small intestines

kerato refers to the cornea

labia lip
lacri refers to the lacrimal duct
lamin refers to the lamina of vertebra
laparo refers to the abdomen
-lapaxy to empty out
laryngo refers to the larynx
lem refers to a sheath around nerves
-lexia refers to reading
lipo refers to fat tissue
-lith stones, such as kidney stones
lobe part of an organ, such as a lung
-lysis dissolution of adhesions

-malacia softness
mammo refers to the breast
maxilla refers to maxillary sinus
meato a passageway or opening
mega large
-megaly indicates largeness
mening refers to the meninges
meno indicates menstruating
metri refers to the uterus
metro measure
myel refers to bone marrow
myo refers to muscle
myring refers to tympanic membrane

naso refers to nasal, nose
neo new
nephro kidney
neur nerve

olecran refers to elbow
oligo small or few
-ologist person who studies a subject
-oma tumor

oophor refers to the ovaries
orch refers to the testicles
oro refers to oral
-osis indicates a disease
osteo bone
ot refers to the ear
-oxia oxygen

palato refers to the palate
-partum refers to labor
patell refers to kneecap
-pathy indicates a disease
peri near or surrounding
-pepsia digestion
-pexy to hold or fasten
phac refers to the lens
-phagia eat
phak refers to the lens
pharyngo refers to pharynx
phlebo refers to veins
-planesis wandering, mobility
-plasty to reconstruct or repair
-plegia stroke or paralysis
pleur surrounding the lungs
-plicatio to fold
-pnea breath
pneumo lungs
pore a tiny opening
post after, behind
procto anus
prosta refers to the prostate
-ptosis dropping
pulmo refers to the lungs
pyel refers to pelvis of kidney
pylor refers to the pylorus

renal refers to the kidney
rhino refers to the nose
-rrhage abnormal or excessive flow or discharge
-rrhea indicates a discharge

-rrhaphy surgical suturing
-rrhexis rupture

salping refers to the ovarian ducts
scapul refers to the shoulder blade
-schisis separation
-scler hard, refers to the sclera
-scope an instrument used to examine a body part
-scopy using a scope to look at a body part
sequestr to separate, isolate
sialo refers to the salivary glands
sigmoido refers to part of the colon
sinu refers to the sinus
-spasm involuntary contraction of an muscle
-spermia refers to sperm
spondyl refers to a vertebra
stape indicates the stapes
-staxis to drip
stea refers to fat
sten narrowing
-stomy a surgical opening
strobo whirling
sub below
supra above
sympathy refers to the sympathetic nervous system
synov refers to synovial membrane

tachy swift, fast
tarsal refers to bones in the foot
-tasis indicates stretching
tendo refers to tendon
teno refers to tendon
thoraco refers to the chest
thrombo refers to a blood clot
thyro refers to the thyroid cartilage
tibi refers to the larger bone in the calf
-tomy a surgical cut

trach refers to the trachea
trachel refers to the neck of a body part
trans through
tympan refers to the tympanic membrane

uln refers to the ulna
ur refers to urine or urinary tract

valv refers to the heart valve
vas refers to the vas deferens
vasculo refers to blood vessels
ven refers to vein
vesico refers to the bladder

-xerosis dryness

zoo refers to animal

Terms, Page

achalasia, 252
adenectomy, 26
adenitis, 24
adenocarcinoma, 28
adenopathy, 26
adenosclerosis, 24
alveoalgia, 217
alveolar process, 208
alveolectomy, 208
alveoloplasty, 217
amniocentesis, 284
anastomosis, 92
aneurysm, 128
angiectomy, 35
angiitis, 30
angina, 28
angiocardiogram, 32

angiocardiography, 35
angiocarditis, 35
angiogram, 35
angiograph, 35
angiography, 35
angioma, 28
angioplasty, 30
angiosclerosis, 28
angiosis, 35
angiostenosis, 134
anomaly, 120
antepartum, 284
antrectomy, 254
antrotomy, 172
antrum, 253
aorta, 127
aortic stenosis, 122
aortoplasty, 134
arteriogram, 8
arteriography, 10
arteriorrhaphy, 8
arteriovenous fistula, 148
arteritis, 10
arthralgia, 40
arthrocele, 139
arthrogram, 51
arthropathy, 20
arthrostomy, 139
arthrotomy, 20
arytenoid, 177
arytenoidectomy, 178
atherosclerosis, 130
athrocentesis, 62
atrial, 120
auricle, 190
azoospermia, 288

biliary tract, 264
bladder, 79
blepharedema, 228
blepharitis, 30

Visit

quicklearnguides.com

for more information, the latest
details and to inquire about quantity
discounts.

Also available:

ICD-10-CM Quick Learn

NOTES...

Made in the USA
Coppell, TX
11 April 2023

15495893R00208